ying
the
ial:
ons
of
difference

social policy: welfare, power and diversity

series editor: john clarke

This book is part of a series produced in association with The Open University. The complete list of books in the series is as follows:

Embodying the Social: Constructions of Difference, edited by Esther Saraga

Forming Nation, Framing Welfare, edited by Gail Lewis

Welfare: Needs, Rights and Risks, edited by Mary Langan

Unsettling Welfare: The Reconstruction of Social Policy, edited by Gordon Hughes and Gail Lewis

Imagining Welfare Futures, edited by Gordon Hughes

The books form part of the Open University course D218 *Social Policy: Welfare, Power and Diversity*. If you would like to study this or any other Open University course, details can be obtained from the Central Enquiries Data Service, PO Box 625, Dane Road, Milton Keynes MK1 1TY. For availability of other course components, contact Open University Worldwide, The Berrill Building, Walton Hall, Milton Keynes MK7 6AA.

embodying the social:
constructions of difference

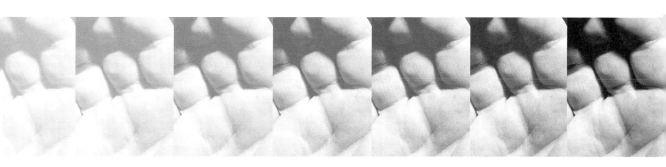

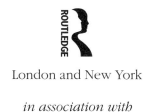

London and New York

in association with

The Open University

edited
by
**esther
saraga**

First published 1998 by Routledge
11 New Fetter Lane, London EC4P 4EE

Simultaneously published in the USA and Canada
by Routledge
29 West 35th Street, New York, NY 10001

The opinions expressed are not necessarily those of the Course Team or of The Open University

Edited, designed and typeset by The Open University
Printed and bound by Scotprint Ltd, Musselburgh, Scotland

British Library Cataloguing in Publication Data
A catalogue record for this book is available from The British Library

Library of Congress Cataloguing in Publication Data
A catalogue record for this book has been requested

ISBN 0-415-18131-3 (hbk)
ISBN 0-415-18132-1 (pbk)

1.1

Contents

Preface

Embodying the Social is the first of five books in a new series of introductory social policy texts published by Routledge in association with The Open University. The series, entitled *Social Policy: Welfare, Power and Diversity*, examines central issues in the study of how social welfare is organized in the UK today. The series is designed to provide a social scientific understanding of the complex and fascinating issues of social welfare in contemporary society. It specifically examines the key issues arising from questions concerning the changing nature of the welfare state and social policy in the UK, giving particular emphasis to the processes of social differentiation and their implications for social welfare. The series also emphasizes the ways in which social problems and solutions to them have been socially constructed and are subject to historical change. More generally, the books use social scientific theories and research studies together with, and in contrast to, other forms of 'knowing' about social welfare and social issues (such as common sense). This is done in order to raise key questions about how society 'works', how social change occurs, and how social order is maintained.

The five books form the core components of an Open University course which shares the title of this series. This first book, *Embodying the Social*, examines the central issue of how patterns of social difference are socially constructed. It traces the implications of such constructions for social policy – for example, the effects of shifting conceptions of disability – and examines their contested character. In exploring these concerns, this first book begins to establish the central focus of the course and series on *diversity*, the formations of *social difference*, and *power*, in particular the power to define our understanding of such differences.

The second book, *Forming Nation, Framing Welfare*, addresses the relationships between nation, state and social welfare by tracing the historical conflicts and constructions that have shaped our modern conceptions of citizenship. The book explores the making of the nation – the inclusions and exclusions of different social groups – and the role of social policy in that process.

The third book, *Welfare: Needs, Rights and Risks*, focuses on a rather different issue, namely the questions of who gets welfare and under what conditions. This book examines how categories of need, desert, risk and rights play a central role in constructing access to welfare, particularly in circumstances where arguments over rationing, priority setting and limited resources are central to the forming of social policies.

The fourth book, *Unsettling Welfare*, deals with the rise and fall of the welfare state in the UK, and traces the ways in which the relationship between social welfare and the state has been reconstructed at the end of the twentieth century. In particular, it focuses on the consequences of the break-up of the political, economic and social settlements that had sustained the 'old' welfare state in the thirty years after the Second World War.

The fifth and final book, *Imagining Welfare Futures*, looks at the prospects for the further remaking of social welfare around the focal points of citizenship, community and consumerism.

Because these books are integral elements of an Open University course, they are designed in distinctive ways in order to contribute to the process of student learning. Each book is constructed as an interactive teaching text, and this has implications for how the book can be read. The chapters form a planned sequence, so that each chapter builds on its predecessors and each concludes with a set of suggestions for further reading in relation to its core topics. The books are also organized around a series of learning processes:

- *Activities*: highlighted in colour, these are exercises which invite you to take an active part in working on the text and are intended to test your understanding and develop reflective analysis.

- *Comments*: these provide feedback from the chapter's author(s) on the activities and enable you to compare your responses with the thoughts of the author(s).

- *Shorter questions*: again highlighted in colour, these are designed to encourage you to pause and reflect on what you have just read.

- *Key words*: these are concepts that play a central role in each chapter and in the course's approach to studying social policy; they are highlighted in colour in the text and in the margins.

While each book in the series is self-contained, there are also references backwards and forwards to the other books. Readers who wish to use the series as the basis for a systematic introduction to studying social policy should note that the references to chapters in other books of the series appear in bold type. The objective of this approach to presenting the material is to enable readers to grasp and reflect on the central themes, issues and arguments not only of each chapter, but also of each book and the series as a whole.

The production of this book and the others that make up the series draws on the expertise of a whole range of people beyond its editors and authors. Each book reflects the combined efforts of an Open University course team: the 'collective teacher' at the heart of The Open University's educational system. Each chapter in these books has been through a process of drafts and comments to refine both its content and its approach to teaching. This process of development leaves us indebted to our consultant authors, our panel of tutor advisers and our course assessor. It also brings together and benefits from a range of other skills – of our secretarial staff, editors, designers, librarians – to translate the ideas into the finished product. All of these activities are held together by the course manager, who ensures that all these component parts and people fit together successfully. Our thanks to them all.

John Clarke

Introduction

by John Clarke and Esther Saraga

Embodying the Social is an introduction to some of the most important – and challenging – issues involved in the study of social policy. How we view the conditions and consequences of social policies depends very heavily on how we understand the society in which such policies are formulated and implemented. At the centre of this problem is the question of how we make sense of patterns of difference between individuals and groups in society. We might ask a number of questions about this issue of difference:

- What sorts of differences are visible in our society?
- What sorts of differences have consequences in our society?
- What do we do about such differences?
- Where do these differences come from?

These questions lead to different tasks for social scientists. The first involves a degree of 'mapping' the society in order to identify what patterns of difference exist (for the social sciences are concerned with patterns rather than individual idiosyncrasies or random occurrences). The second of these questions also involves this sense of 'mapping' the society, but this time it involves searching for evidence of the consequences of these patterned differences. Do differences mean that people are treated differently? Do the differences result in unequal opportunities or outcomes for people? Do the differences have an effect on people's life chances: their educational, occupational, financial, familial or health prospects? Some differences, in other words, make a difference.

The third question has historically been the primary focus of social policy as an area of academic enquiry. It has been concerned with the possibilities, policies and consequences of social action intended to remedy, control or improve particular social conditions. For example, the earliest objectives of social policies in this country, outlined in the Poor Law, were addressed to concerns such as what to do with those who could not support themselves – the impoverished, elderly or disabled people who were unable to make a living. The difference addressed was the difference between the normal, able-bodied, employable population and those who, for one reason or another, could not or would not earn their livelihood.

If we look back over this description of the concerns of the Poor Law, it is possible to see why the fourth question is so important to the study of social policy, and why it is the focus of this book. What sorts of differences were being addressed in the Poor Law, and how are those differences understood or explained? When terms like the 'normal, able-bodied and employable' are juxtaposed to 'the impoverished, elderly or disabled' we are dealing with the consequences of processes of social construction. These divisions are not natural, inevitable or intrinsic to the people being so described. They are the result of ways of thinking about, defining and interpreting the social world. 'Employability' (or the lack of it) is a social characteristic rather than a personal attribute. It sums up a variety of social judgements about what sorts of people make desirable employees, and these judgements change over time and between societies.

1

These issues form the core of *Embodying the Social*. The construction of difference is a necessary starting-point for the study of social policy because how differences are constructed – the way that they are made to mean something – is the basis from which decisions about social policies flow. How we define or interpret a pattern of difference has profound consequences for how it is acted upon. For example, if we view unemployment as a result of personal failings, we will react to it in a different way than if we see it as the result of economic mismanagement on a national or international scale.

This book is called *Embodying the Social* because the social constructions of difference that it addresses are ones that work in a particular way – they are constructions that speak of the 'natural' basis of the differences in question. A whole range of differences in British and other societies are represented as being the result of natural, biological or body-based distinctions. Thus the different social roles, opportunities and inequalities between men and women have long been accounted for by reference to the divergent biological capacities of men and women. In this book, this 'naturalizing' process of social construction is examined in relation to other patterns of difference. What they have in common is that the construction of a basis in nature explains away social processes and affects the way social policies address these differences. Chapter 1, by John Clarke and Allan Cochrane, introduces this way of thinking about the socially constructed nature of differences and its implications for studying social problems and social policy. Chapters 2, 3 and 4 by Gordon Hughes, Gail Lewis and Esther Saraga draw out this analysis by examining how particular patterns of difference have been constructed. These chapters highlight two extremely important issues – first, the ways in which some differences are 'naturalized' and, second, the existence of competing or conflicting constructions of social differences. There is rarely one unchallenged construction of such patterns of difference. The final chapter by Esther Saraga reviews the arguments of the book, drawing out central themes and issues.

Finally, if you look back over this introduction you will find a number of words or phrases enclosed in quotation marks – for example, 'impoverished, elderly or disabled'. This is a stylistic device closely associated with the perspective that this book takes on the social construction of differences. It is used as a short-hand way of indicating that the words bracketed in this way are themselves social constructions rather than naturally occurring patterns or characteristics. So, 'disabled' here abbreviates a phrase that if written out in full would read 'the group of people that our society currently conventionally categorizes as disabled and therefore treats as different from the norm of being able-bodied'. This use of quotation marks often irritates readers, but we hope that indicating how long the sentences might get if authors did not adopt this convention will make its advantages clear.

CHAPTER I

The Social Construction of Social Problems

by John Clarke and Allan Cochrane

Contents

1   Introduction

In this chapter we explore the question of what it is that makes social problems *social*. What is it that makes some issues and not others worthy of public attention, anxiety or action? The emphasis in this chapter is placed on examining the processes by which social problems are *socially constructed*. We will be concerned with the ways in which problems are identified, defined, given meaning and acted upon. In the course of examining these processes, we will be giving particular attention to the significance of *conflicts* about how social problems are defined, interpreted and responded to. These issues about the social construction of social problems form the central concerns of this chapter and provide the basis for exploring a number of approaches in the social sciences that address these processes of defining, interpreting and giving meaning to social problems.

2   What is 'social' about a social problem?

In the late twentieth century a list of current social problems in the UK might include poverty, homelessness, child abuse, disaffected young people and non-attendance at school, school discipline, the treatment of vulnerable people in institutional care, vandalism, road rage, lone parenting and divorce. This brief list was drawn up from news items on television and radio and in newspapers in the month that this chapter was being written. As you read this chapter, some of these may still be issues, some may have disappeared, while new problems may have attracted attention. It is not obvious what they have in common, except that they are the subject of current concern. That fact – the capturing of public interest, anxiety or concern – is probably the best place to start this discussion, since it suggests that one answer to what is 'social' about a social problem is that such problems have gained a hold on the attention of a particular society at a particular time.

There is a point in stressing the word 'particular' here. Other societies may be preoccupied by other problems: what commands public attention in Germany, the USA or China is likely to be different in at least some respects to what is a current social problem in the UK. It is also true that if we looked back at earlier historical periods, only some of the list of current social problems would be visible then. In the late nineteenth century, for example, we would find that poverty, the maltreatment of children and divorce were being discussed as social problems, but others on the list did not attract much attention. There are two possible explanations for such differences. One is that social problems change. If in the late nineteenth century there were no homeless people, then we would not expect homelessness to have been discussed as a social problem. The second reason is that what is perceived as a social problem may change. Thus there may indeed have been people who were homeless in the late nineteenth century, but their situation was perceived not as a social problem, but rather as a 'fact of life' or as the consequence of mere individual misfortune – neither of which would make it a *social* problem.

Writing in the 1950s, the American sociologist C. Wright Mills (1959, pp.7–10) drew a distinction between 'personal troubles' and 'public issues'. He suggested that although there were many 'troubles' or 'problems' that individuals experienced in their lives, not all of these emerged as 'public issues' which commanded public interest and attention or which were seen as requiring public responses ('what can we do about X?'). Mills's use of the term 'personal' may be slightly misleading, since it implies that it is the difference between individual and collective experience that matters. For us, however, the important distinction is between issues that are 'private' (that is, to be handled within households, families or even communities) and those which are 'public' (that is, to be handled through forms of social intervention or regulation). One factor that may make a difference to whether things are perceived as private troubles or public issues is scale or volume. If only a few people experience some form of trouble, then it is likely to remain a private matter and not attract public concern. If, however, large numbers of people begin to experience this same trouble – or fear they might – it may become a public issue. The process can probably best be explored with the help of an example.

2.1 From private trouble to public issue: the emergence of negative equity

In the housing market, owner-occupiers have occasionally sold their property at a price below that which they paid for it. In the early 1990s, large numbers of property owners in the UK (and particularly in south-east England) found that the market value of their houses and flats had fallen below the original purchase price. A private trouble emerged as a public issue. It was named, and became the problem of 'negative equity'. This was identified as a widespread problem rather than a matter of individual misfortune: it was seen to have causes (in the state of the economy) which lay beyond the reach of the individual. It was also identified as something that required a public response – from mortgage lenders and the government.

Can this shift of a private trouble to a public issue be understood as a consequence of the numbers of people involved?

The numbers involved provide only part of the explanation why this trouble became a public issue. Other 'troubles' involving equally large numbers of people attracted less attention and concern. For example, the continuing rise in rents for tenants of council housing and housing associations, which took place at the same time, was largely viewed as a fact of life. Furthermore, despite the attempts of housing professionals to place the issue on the public agenda, the decaying state of Britain's owner-occupied housing stock (built before 1945) continued to be defined as a personal problem facing those who happened to be living in older houses. They were expected to resolve it through their own investment in renewal and repair, rather than through any collective effort. We might suggest that a number of other features of negative equity helped it become a public issue:

- *Who was involved?* The social and political standing of those experiencing this trouble affected its visibility. Home owners were seen as innocent victims of a situation beyond their control. They were the symbolic representations of government policies designed to create a 'property-owning democracy'. Negative equity was thus a politically sensitive matter.

- *What was its claim on public attention?* Negative equity was seen as connected to matters of public policy – first, the drive to extend home ownership and, second, the contemporary management of the national economy which was associated with an initial boom and then a slump in housing prices.

- *What sort of problem was it?* Negative equity was seen as having significant social and economic consequences. It was associated with mounting personal debt, a lack of social mobility, and a fear of the future that prevented people taking risks. In particular, it was seen as causing a problem of consumer confidence: this reduced patterns of consumer spending, which in turn further threatened the prospects of economic growth. It was therefore also a political problem for the government, as it provoked extensive public discussion about the presence or absence of a 'feel-good factor', particularly among the government's erstwhile supporters.

What this brief example suggests is that the scale of a 'trouble' is not by itself a sufficient condition for understanding why the trouble becomes a public issue. We need to understand the social context in which it occurs – its links to other current issues and values. The case of negative equity also suggests that we need to think about who is involved and how they are perceived, in terms of their social standing and significance. In very simple terms, we might suggest that there are two routes to troubles becoming public issues which are distinguished by the question: *whose problem is this?*

Some troubles become social or public problems as a result of the actions of those people who experience them (or those who speak on behalf of such people). Thus, campaigns aim to capture public attention and direct it to the conditions or experiences that specific groups of people are suffering. Negative equity would be one example of this route. Other examples include campaigns to draw attention to the widespread incidence of domestic violence, despite its relative public invisibility; to raise concern about the abuse or maltreatment of vulnerable people in institutional care; or to reveal the scale of, and suffering associated with, homelessness. Such campaigns try to articulate the experience of a particular condition and demand public action to remedy it. This route is built around the argument that people *have* problems.

The second route is different, in that it is built around the argument that some people *are* problems. There are some types of people who are seen as a problem for others or for society at large (even if these people do not define themselves in the same way). For example, we might be able to identify groups of people who are seen to pose a threat or danger to society in some way: vandals, noisy neighbours, hooligans, prostitutes, the mentally ill, and so on. The demand here is that society does something about 'these people' – police them, lock them up, treat them, and so forth.

Sometimes, of course, the same problem might be identified through both these routes. If we examine homelessness as a social problem, it is possible to see its being defined as a problem that some people have and as a problem that some people are. In the first case, the problem is perceived as the lack of access to a basic human need – adequate accommodation – which results in homeless people experiencing deprivation, misery and suffering. The appeal is to a sense of social justice. In the second case, the problem of homelessness is perceived as a threat to everyday life: homeless people clutter city streets, are a health risk, prevent 'normal' people going about their daily business, and are associated with crime and other perceived threats to the rest of society. The appeal is to a sense of social order. Both routes acknowledge the importance of social differentiation, but they do so in different ways. The first implies that steps need to be taken to reverse or compensate for the inequalities or unfairness that arises from particular social arrangements, while the second implies that those who do not conform to accepted and widely understood norms – or standards – of behaviour need to be taught or helped to do so.

social justice

social order

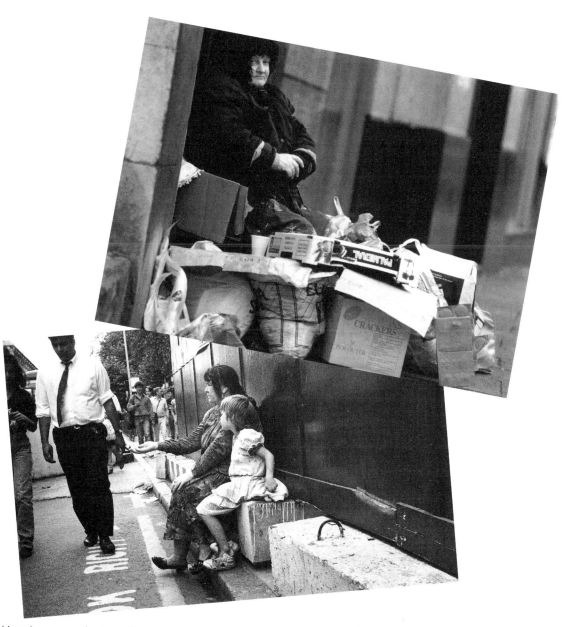

Homelessness: a shortage of adequate accommodation, or a threat to society?

Can you think of other social problems where both these routes are visible?

Use the grid below to help you to do this. We have taken one example, 'the mentally ill', and have filled in the first column to show you how you might answer. Try to fill in the second column, and then see if you can add two further examples.

Social problem	People *have* problems	People *are* problems
Mental illness	Mentally ill people are ill through no fault of their own and require/deserve treatment. Mental illness can affect all of us (and even if we have not all suffered from it in some form, most of us will know someone who has). As far as possible mentally ill people should be re-integrated into their communities, since excluding them from ordinary life is likely to make their condition worse.	

2.2 Social problems and social policy

Whether social problems emerge as issues of social justice or social order, they are usually associated with the idea that 'something must be done'. Social problems represent conditions that should not be allowed to continue because they are perceived to be problems for society, requiring society to react to them and find remedies. Where private troubles are matters for the individuals involved to resolve, public issues or social problems demand a public response. The range of possible public responses is, of course, very wide. At one extreme we might point to interventions that are intended to suppress or control social problems: locking people up, inflicting physical punishments or deprivations on them, even – in the most severe form – killing them. Such interventions are intended to stop social problems by means of controlling the people who are seen as problems (juvenile delinquents, drug takers, thieves, terrorists). Those who seek the suppression and control of social problems are usually, but not always, associated with the view that social problems are a challenge or threat to social order. The point about 'not always' is important, since sometimes these types of intervention are presented not in terms of protecting society or social order, but as being in 'the best interests' of the person being punished or 'treated': they need a 'bit of discipline', they respect 'toughness', and so on.

However, other interventions are intended to remedy or improve the circumstances or social conditions that cause problems – bringing about greater social justice, enhancing social welfare, or providing a degree of social protection. Thus, the development of welfare states in most advanced industrial societies during the twentieth century was associated with attempts to remedy social problems or to provide citizens with some collective protection from dangers to their economic and social well-being. In the process, a whole range of issues moved from being private troubles to becoming matters of public concern and intervention. Between the late nineteenth and the mid twentieth centuries, these societies redefined the distinction between private and public matters. Sending children to school became a matter of public compulsion rather than the private parental choice that it had been until the middle of the nineteenth century. Health became a focus of public finance, provision and intervention rather than being left to private arrangements. For most of the nineteenth century unemployment was seen as something that people chose (by refusing to take work), while for most of the twentieth century it has been seen as something against which collective action and defence by the state was necessary. Unemployment was not a social problem in the UK for most of the nineteenth century, although the unemployed themselves were certainly seen as a threat to social order (being beggars, thieves and a bad example to other workers).

In the process, citizens in advanced industrial societies came to associate social problems with social interventions – often involving action by the state – that were intended to reform or ameliorate the conditions that created problems. Social welfare, and the welfare state in particular, was intimately linked to social problems. The attempts to remedy social problems – combating illness, poverty or homelessness – drove the growth of the welfare state during the twentieth century. But the questions of whether these issues really are social problems and whether state welfare is the best remedy have reappeared towards the end of the twentieth century (see, for example, **Lewis and Hughes, 1998**). There are now echoes of the nineteenth-century arguments that many social problems are 'really' private troubles and not public issues, and therefore should not need social intervention by public agencies. The revival of such arguments is an important reminder that one central aspect of what is 'social' about social problems is the way in which these problems are socially perceived, defined and comprehended.

Different private troubles become defined as social problems in particular societies and in specific periods through a complex process of social construction. Social construction implies an active process of definition and redefinition in which some issues are widely understood to be social problems, while others are not. Just because unemployment was identified as a social problem – or public trouble – in the middle of the twentieth century, that does not mean that it will always be defined in this way. Even if unemployment

social construction

remains defined as a social problem, it is not necessarily the case that the *nature* of the problem will always be understood in the same way. A move from the notion that unemployed people *have* problems to the idea that unemployed people *are* problems has major implications for the direction of public policy. If unemployment is understood as a problem created by a wider economic failure, then an appropriate policy response might be both to attempt to revitalize the economy in order to create jobs and to provide financial support in the meantime. If, however, unemployment is perceived to arise from either a failure of the unemployed to seek employment or the lack of necessary skills among unemployed people, then an appropriate policy response might be to discourage people from relying on state-provided income support (for example by reducing levels of benefit and introducing stricter rules on entitlement) and to encourage them to participate in relevant skills training. Since the mid 1980s in the UK there has been a marked shift in emphasis from the first to the second approach.

Summary

We have seen that social problems are 'social' in the sense that they capture public attention. They are more than private troubles, perhaps through reasons of scale but certainly because they are able to connect with other public issues, values and concerns – for example, with contemporary concerns about social justice or social order. They are historically and culturally specific – that is, they belong to, or are visible in, particular societies at particular times. Finally, while they may be associated with changing social conditions (a rise or fall in the numbers of people in a particular condition such as poverty or homelessness), their status as social problems depends upon how they are *perceived*. If, for example, a condition such as homelessness is seen as a matter of individual choice or misfortune, it is unlikely to be viewed as a 'social' problem requiring public attention and action. A process of social construction determines both which issues are defined as social problems and the ways in which they are defined as such.

3 'What everybody knows': common sense and social problems

This concern with social construction may seem troubling or even a distraction from the real business of studying social problems. However, it is built on one of the starting points of the social scientific approach, namely that in order to study society we must distance ourselves from what we already know about it. We need to become 'strangers' in a world that is familiar. The defining characteristic of a 'stranger' is that she or he does not know those things which we take for granted. Strangers require the 'obvious' to be explained to them. In doing social science, then, there is a need to stand back from what we already know or believe and be distanced from, or sceptical about, those things which 'everybody knows'. Let us go back to the list of current social problems mentioned at the start of the chapter and look in more detail at the issue of poverty. What is it that 'everybody knows' about poverty in our society?

Make your own list here of 'what everybody knows' about poverty and then compare it with ours overleaf.

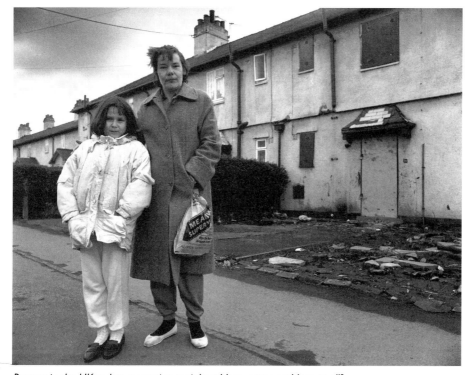

Poverty in the UK today: a growing social problem, or no problem at all?

Our list of 'what everybody knows' is as follows:

- There is no real poverty in Britain today.
- There are more people living in poverty now than in the 1970s.
- Nobody needs to be poor.
- Some people would be poor no matter how much you helped them.
- Poor parents produce poor children.
- There are too many people in jobs with low wages.
- People wouldn't be poor if they knew how to manage better.
- Poverty acts as a spur to try hard.
- Government polices have made the rich richer and the poor poorer.
- People have become too dependent on state hand-outs.
- People are stuck in poverty traps.
- There will always be people who won't help themselves.

■ ■ ■

We have seen or heard all of these statements in the last two years. Each of them has been announced with the certainty of truth. 'What everybody knows' turns out to be simultaneously over-simplified, complicated and contradictory. Each statement constructs the problem of poverty in a different way and implies different types of causes. One contribution that social scientists are expected to make is to say, 'well, that may be what you think, but the real facts are these …'. It is, however, not quite so easy. One reason for this is that defining poverty is itself a contested issue – should it mean an *absolute* lack of resources or should it be measured *relative* to the standards of the particular society? Even if agreement could be found on the definition, this still leaves open the issue of how to interpret or explain those 'facts'.

An alternative starting point is to examine how poverty is socially constructed as a problem – to scrutinize 'what everybody knows', alongside public, political and policy definitions of the problem and to disentangle the constructions that we find. This means that the practice of social science involves what we might call 'systematic scepticism' – distancing oneself from the 'common-sense' understandings.

Let us turn back to our list of statements about poverty and see if we can identify some of the key features of how poverty is socially constructed in the UK today. The first striking feature is that there are conflicting definitions about whether or not poverty is a current social problem. Those who view poverty as meaning an absolute lack of resources can see no problem: poverty simply does not exist in the UK (although it may do in other parts of the world). Such a view is contested by those who define poverty in relative terms and argue that poverty has, in fact, increased – for them it is a growing social problem. This suggests that 'poverty' is not simply a matter of academic definition but is at the centre of conflicting social understandings about whether people are 'really', 'truly' or 'genuinely' poor. If we believe they are not, there is no social problem which requires attention or any social response. This is the first, and simplest, split in common-sense (and political) debate about poverty: is it a social problem or not?

The second striking feature of these 'everybody knows' statements is that they evoke widely divergent views of poor people and the causes of poverty. This common sense about poverty is contradictory and contested. Some people look to the 'external' causes of poverty – the social, economic and political conditions that make some people poor. Others look to the 'internal' causes of poverty – the attitudes, behaviours or morals that lead some people to make themselves poor. What is noticeable is that even brief statements such as 'nobody needs to be poor' carry a set of unspoken assumptions about the nature of society and the nature of poverty. 'Nobody needs to be poor' tells us that:

- We live in a society of opportunities for everyone.
- There are no external conditions that force people to be poor.
- If people are poor, then this is something to do with the choices they make.
- Therefore poverty is the result of poor people making bad choices (in how they live, work, spend money, etc.).

A short, five-word statement contains a series of assumptions which add up to a theory of society (an 'opportunity' society), a theory of human behaviour (people make choices) and an explanation of poverty (some people make bad choices). It also implies how the rest of society should position itself in relation to poverty: it is not 'our' responsibility if 'they' make bad choices. Nor is there anything 'we' can do about it (except perhaps educate 'them' to make better choices). Each of the statements above could be assessed in this way, exploring the assumptions about society, behaviour and poverty that underpin them. The same approach could be applied to statements about other social problems.

ACTIVITY 1.3

If we were to consider discussions which focus on lone-parent families as a social problem, we would find ourselves confronted with comments like 'the rising numbers of single mothers indicate a moral crisis'. What assumptions do you think underlie this statement?

COMMENT

We would list the following assumptions, but you may have noted others:

- There is a group of people who are single mothers (rather than different types of single mothers, for example widowed, divorced, separated, never married).
- There used to be a moral order – a system of values, norms and ideas that prevented single motherhood.
- Something has changed to undermine that moral order (explanations of this may vary – we have become less religious; people are more concerned with individual freedom; there has been a rise in permissiveness; welfare systems have provided benefits to lone parents, making it easier to choose to be a lone parent).
- A crisis exists, and all crises need something to be done about them (in this case, some means of restoring traditional family values or morality).

■ ■ ■

One thing that a social science approach can do, by taking the perspective of the stranger, is to examine the content of common-sense statements about social problems and question the assumptions on which they are based. In the next section we will look further at the sorts of assumptions and explanations that are put to work in the different common-sense views of poverty. However, we want now to note a few other features of such views (we shall return to these later in this chapter as well as in other chapters).

The statements about poverty that we started with are not just random or throwaway thoughts that people express on the spur of the moment. They are social claims, each one implying that we all share the assumptions contained within the statements (even though the assumptions are profoundly different and even contradictory). 'Common sense', used as a term to describe such statements of 'what everybody knows', directs our attention as social scientists to the underlying theories, perspectives and assumptions that are mobilized through simple statements and claims. A society's stock of common sense can therefore be seen as a repository or storeroom of bits of knowledge on which people can draw in discussing society and its problems. One task for a social science approach is therefore to make an inventory of this repository – to catalogue the bits and pieces of knowledge that people can and do draw on. If, for example, we were to go back to the issue of lone parents, we would need to take stock of the other possible elements of common sense that are available when lone parents are discussed. In addition to moral crisis, we might need to catalogue views about the irresponsibility of men, the changing pressures on family life, the causes of changes in divorce and marriage, and whether the same sorts of explanations apply to widowed, separated and never married women – as well as to lone fathers.

If we pursue this idea of common sense as a repository a little further, we can see another task for a social science analysis. The stock of this repository has been built up over time, having been deposited by previous generations and added to over time. It is not simply 'what we think today', but has a history. One thing we can do, then, is to look for the 'traces' of older ideas, to see how they are recirculated and kept alive across decades and even centuries. For example, ideas about the difference between the 'deserving' and 'undeserving' poor are deposits from mid-nineteenth-century discussions (and policies) about the problem of poverty. They reflect anxieties of that time about how to deal with poor people, and how to ensure that social policies – the provision of benefits by the state or by charitable sources – did not go to the 'wrong sort of people'. Such ideas, together with their assumptions about society and human behaviour, were not just dumped in a dark corner of the storeroom and left to accumulate dust, never to be seen again. Rather, they are brought out again from time to time and threaded into new issues and debates, for example about whether we should have universal benefits or ones that are targeted at the 'most needy' or about how to distinguish between 'scroungers' and those 'genuinely' in need. Ideas about people getting their 'just deserts' and the moral worth of different people have been a recurrent feature of discussions about poverty in the UK.

Finally, it is important to note that this approach to common sense is not merely an academic exercise, in the sense of being of no practical use or interest. Taking an inventory of common sense and examining the continuing traces of past ideas and the ways in which they are revived and used are an integral part of the study of social problems and social policies. There are three aspects which make an understanding of common sense an essential feature of studying social problems:

1   Each 'bit' of common sense involves a claim to be the truth: for example, statements about poverty are not just different, but are contested in conflicts where each position (and its assumptions and consequences) seeks to be 'what everybody knows'. Part of the approach to social science is not just to 'take an inventory' but to ask which strands are currently the dominant or most widely accepted ones, and how this pattern can be explained.

2   Common-sense views are not just discussions or conversations that take place in idle moments. They are also connected to social and political action. Political parties address bits of common sense in their efforts to persuade people that they have the right answers and that their policies should be implemented. Indeed, one of the most potent claims made by political parties is that they are on the side of 'common sense' or that what they are proposing is merely 'what everybody knows'. If we have taken an inventory of common sense, we are in a position to ask: which part of common sense is being addressed here, and what has happened to the other parts?

3   These connections – the dominance of some ideas over others, and the political articulation of some ideas – matter, because they lead to social action. The predominant definition of poverty, explanation of its causes, or view of who is 'deserving', has consequences, for these shape how the society and its political institutions respond to poverty.

We shall return to these aspects of common sense in section 6.1 and in the following chapters.

Summary

Social scientists need to stand back, to view common sense or 'what everybody knows' from the perspective of a stranger. Common sense about social problems such as poverty involves a process of social construction, drawing on a repository or storeroom of underlying theories and assumptions. Common sense has been built up over time, carrying with it traces of earlier understandings which are also brought into discussions of new issues and debates. Common sense is itself divided, reflecting contested and conflicting claims about the nature of society and social problems. Although we have talked here of different 'bits' of common sense, some authors prefer to talk about a range of common *senses* (that is, in the plural). You will find that later chapters in this book use this formulation. In discussions of social problems, each position seeks to be 'what everybody knows' – the dominant common sense. This has direct consequences for the development of social policy through political initiatives. The sceptical analysis of common sense is, therefore, of practical as well as academic importance.

4   Tracing the deposits: competing explanations of social problems

If we can agree that poverty is a social problem, we are led to another question: what sort of social problem is it? For some, it is a social problem because people should not be poor: it involves social injustice. For others, poverty is a social problem because poor people behave badly (or bring up children poorly): it involves social disorder. We therefore have another parting of the ways, with some believing that social justice requires poor people to become less poor, and others believing that poor people need to be made better people. In part, this split between justice and order reflects different common-sense views of why poor people are poor. We would suggest that it is possible to see at least three different conceptions of the causes of poverty underlying the list of comments following Activity 1.2: poverty is natural/inevitable; poverty is the result of poor people; poverty is the result of economic and/or political causes.

4.1   Poverty as natural/inevitable

There is a construction of poverty that identifies it as a necessary feature of social life: some people will be better endowed, try harder or be more successful than others, and inequality will be an inevitable result (see, for example, Herrnstein and Murray, 1994, who argue that low levels of intelligence are the main determinants of poverty in the USA). Interfering with this natural order of things is dangerous, particularly because it prevents poverty acting as a spur to try harder. This is the basis of the American economist George Gilder's attack on 'welfare culture', his term for state programmes intended to diminish the impact of poverty:

> The most serious fraud is committed not by the members of the welfare culture but by the creators of it, who conceal from the poor, both adults and children, the most fundamental realities of their lives: that to live well and escape poverty they will have to keep their families together at all costs and will have to work harder than the classes above them. In order to succeed the poor need most of all the spur of their poverty.
>
> (Gilder, 1981, p.118)

In this perspective, poverty is simultaneously natural and socially necessary. Inequalities are both the natural result of unequal performance in a competitive world and necessary to keep people trying to succeed. The response to the problem of poverty is to try to restore it to its 'natural' state, since programmes designed to ameliorate it prevent people trying to succeed. As a result, poor people become 'dependent' on welfare benefits and 'demoralized', losing the moral urge to fend for themselves and their families.

4.2   Poverty as the result of poor people

The second cluster of common-sense ideas about poverty centre around the theme that the character and behaviour of some types of people causes them to be poor. Such people are in some way 'flawed'. There may, of course, be different types of flaw, but poor people are distinguished from the rest of 'us' by some characteristic that makes 'them' poor. This might be their moral character (they are lazy, shiftless, workshy); it might be their abilities or capacities (they cannot budget properly); or it might be that they have not been properly socialized (they have not learnt the value of hard work, thrift, etc.).

What is the argument in the following quotation?

Such problems – problems of morals, attitude, behaviour – are not susceptible to a quick fix by social policy … If incompetent shopping is the problem, larger hand-outs will not cure it. Higher subsidies will not reform bad budgeting. Whatever the behaviour cause, be it isolation, lack of parental example in domestic economy, illiteracy, poor motivation, depression, self-indulgent or incompetent expenditure by husband, those husbands selfishly not handing enough over to their wives, a failure to look beyond today, simply increasing social security expenditure will not solve it.

(Anderson, 1991, p.27)

COMMENT

Two things are being argued here. One is that there is a range of behaviours and attitudes that create poverty (from poor budgeting to selfish patterns of spending). The other is that these are counterposed to suggested solutions to poverty (increased social security expenditure), which, the author suggests, fail to address the causes that he has identified. Particular definitions of problems often proceed by this dual approach – establishing their own line of argument and rejecting others. They do so because 'what we know about poverty' is not a simple or self-evident set of truths all of which point in the same direction. Poverty – like other social problems – is caught up in multiple definitions and perspectives, each of which tries to claim for itself the status of truth.

■ ■ ■

To return to this particular perspective, it identifies the causes of poverty in the behaviour, attitudes and morals of the poor. They are separated from 'normal' people by these flaws or failings. To stop being poor, they need to become more like the rest of 'us'. This differentiation between the normal and others – sometimes described as deviant – is a recurrent feature of how social problems are talked about, both in 'everyday' language and in academic analyses. Both are concerned to find the factor or 'flaw' that distinguishes the normal from the abnormal. These issues are discussed further in the different contexts of disability, 'race' and sexuality in the following chapters.

deviant

normal/ abnormal

4.3 Poverty as the effect of economic or political causes

The third and final cluster of ideas about poverty are those which imply causes that lie in the external world of the economy and politics. For example, an increase in the number of people working in low-paid jobs produces lower incomes and more people living in relative poverty, or changes in government policy on welfare benefits might reduce incomes or trap people in poverty because they lose benefits when they earn income. These definitions locate poverty as an effect of causes beyond individuals or families – what we might call 'structural' or 'social' causes because they are located in social structures or arrangements that are outside the individual's control. Here is one such argument:

> The poverty of low wages and poor working conditions is often still a hidden factor in the poverty debate. Recent government policies have specifically weakened employment rights ... Alongside the deregulation of employment law, new patterns of employment have changed the profile of the workforce. There has been a marked increase in self-employment and in part-time and low-paid work and a small increase in temporary work. Women are more likely to be in both part-time and temporary work. Many of these jobs are low paid with few employment and social security rights which not only creates poverty, but also stores it up for the future.
>
> (Oppenheim, 1993, p.59)

Although this says things about the people living in poverty (for example, that women are likely to be affected by low-paid and poorly protected employment), it does not treat poverty as being the result of the intrinsic characteristics of such groups but rather as the consequence of economic and political arrangements.

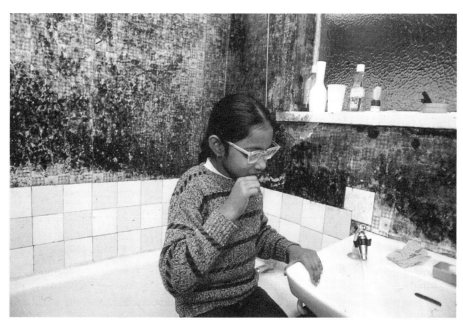

Is poverty a necessary feature of society, the result of inadequate socialization, or the consequence of economic or political arrangements?

4.4   Social science approaches

So far we have looked at three more developed discussions of some of the basic propositions about poverty that we considered in section 3. These three examples could be multiplied: there is a variety of explanations of poverty that we could have used. However, these three allow us to reflect a little on the relationship between social science discussions of social problems and common-sense understandings. It is worth starting with some of the differences.

■   Even these brief extracts from books and articles indicate that social scientists take longer to say things than the rather pithy common-sense statements that we looked at earlier. Cynics might say that this is simply evidence of social scientists being long-winded, but we believe that there is something else involved here. In each case, what is being presented is an *argument*, rather than an *assertion*. Put simply, the authors are trying to set out a series of connections which explain why one thing is connected to or causes another. They make explicit what are implicit in the common-sense statements. In particular, they make explicit causal claims about why poverty occurs.   **causal claims**

■   On the other hand, these are still arguments. The difference between social science and common sense is not an absolute divide between 'opinion' and 'science', where science guarantees truth (and opinion is necessarily incorrect). We have here three social scientists – and we could have had many more – with very different perspectives on the problem of poverty. While each of them would like to have their explanations seen as the truth, none of them can be certified as the truth merely by virtue of their being written by a social scientist. As with common sense, social science is characterized by competing and contested perspectives.   **competing and contested perspectives**

■   Social science approaches also raise the question of evidence. Although the brief extracts that we have used above do not present statistical data or other sorts of information, they nevertheless raise the possibility in different ways. Gilder's argument that 'to escape poverty' the poor need to keep their families together could be tested against some sort of empirical evidence: for example, is there evidence that families with divorced or separated parents are unable to 'escape' poverty? We could probably all think of examples of such families. At the time of writing, parts of the British royal family are undergoing divorce and separation, and it seems unlikely that the children of these marriages will be thrust into poverty. However, one-off examples are not necessarily the same as statistical trends, where lone parenthood appears to be associated with family poverty. Such evidence might vindicate Gilder's argument, but it may also be explained by other perspectives.   **evidence**

In the rest of this chapter we want to distinguish between a social science *approach* and social science *perspectives*. There is a wide variety of different perspectives within the social sciences, providing different theories to explain social phenomena. Some of these emphasize individual characteristics or choices, some stress familial patterns, while others draw attention to structural or societal conditions and processes. These are the competing perspectives or theories. But there is also an issue about how to approach the study of social problems. Throughout this book the emphasis is on examining the diverse ways in which social problems are socially constructed – the ways in which they are defined, understood, made sense of within society. These social constructions may be in the form of common-sense knowledges, political ideologies, or social science perspectives, but they all contribute to the shaping of how social problems are constructed. A central issue for a social science approach, then, is the work of deconstructing them – making them strange rather than obvious, and examining their assumptions about society, people and problems.   **deconstruction**

Summary

Three explanations of poverty developed by social scientists have been considered. The first sees poverty as natural or inevitable, the second focuses on the behaviour of poor people, while the third analyses poverty as the result of economic or political processes. Considering these explanations makes it possible to draw some conclusions about the social science approach to social problems:

- It relies on arguments making causal claims, rather than assertion.
- Social science is characterized by competing and contested perspectives.
- Social scientists use evidence of various sorts to support and explore the arguments they develop; their conclusions can be judged against that evidence.

5 Mapping the field: competing constructions

5.1 Natural/social

In the previous section we looked at the issue of competing explanations of social problems. Here we want to take a rather different approach by starting from one of the major dividing lines between different types of explanation. These dividing lines are ones that recur in the definition, interpretation and explanation of a range of social issues: for example, patterns of inequality between men and women; crime and juvenile delinquency; the persistence of poverty, and so on. Despite the fact that we have referred to these topics as *social* issues or *social* problems, the most basic dividing line between different social constructions is the distinction between the natural and the social. This might seem slightly confusing, given our focus here on social issues, but ideas about the natural basis of social arrangements or social problems are widespread. There are many claims about social issues that begin with the formulation 'It's only natural that …'. For example, it's only natural that 'men go out to work', 'boys will be boys', 'people will not trust other races', and so on.

If we consider this approach as a 'social construction' – a way of perceiving or understanding the world – instead of exploring it in ways which seek to challenge or confirm the 'facts' on which it is based, what effect would that have?

Ideas about the natural basis of society or of social problems within society refer us to a set of claims about the universal laws of biology or evolution that determine how we might behave. Such ideas often place an emphasis on competition, conflict and struggles for evolutionary success (the 'survival of the fittest'). They identify a range of attributes as the biological basis of human society and often insist that these are unchanging and unchangeable. In claims about the natural, biological attributes are often brought forward as explanations of social patterns. Thus, biological differences between men and women are drawn upon to explain differences in social behaviour or patterns of social inequality. Classically, women's biological capacity to bear children (whether they do so in practice or not) has been held to account for a range of social patterns. For example, for many years women's exclusion from education was justified on the grounds that they didn't need to know anything beyond being a wife and mother, because stimulation of the brain would drain energy that should be devoted to the tasks of reproduction. Equally, men's behaviour has been interpreted as the product of biological forces and drives. For instance, biologists have developed an approach known as 'parental investment theory' to explain why women are monogamous home-builders while men are philandering adulterers. According to this theory, the different 'investments' which eggs and sperm represent for the two sexes, produces a different orientation to the genetic challenge of reproduction. Women invest qualitatively (the best chance for a small number of eggs), while men invest quantitatively (scattering their seed). Such distinctions between men and women have been held to account for a variety of social differences – in attitudes, behaviour, sexuality, patterns of employment, levels of income, involvement in politics, and so on (see Chapter 4; also Barash, 1981; Wilson, 1981).

While there are many arguments about whether there is evidence to support this sort of explanation, our main concern with it here is as a distinctive type of social construction. It centres on the claim that our social world is formed and constrained by a variety of natural causes and conditions. The emphasis on the natural in this form of social construction provides a strong claim to authority and truth, by referring to a world of natural laws that are seen as universal and immutable. As a consequence, many of the social constructions that refer to natural conditions or causes tend to warn against attempts to change or tamper with these natural laws. Social 'interference' – for example, attempts to promote greater equality between men and women – is likely to have undesirable and 'unnatural' consequences.

Where social constructions that centre on 'nature' tend to be resistant to change, social constructions that centre on the 'social' conditions and causes of social issues tend to imply the possibility of change, reform or improvement. An emphasis on the social character of social arrangements suggests that such patterns might be re-arranged. Thus, if some forms of undesirable behaviour – such as delinquent behaviour by young men – are defined as resulting from following bad examples, this construction implies that the provision of better role models would lead to improved behaviour. By contrast, 'natural' constructions would draw attention to the biological or genetic basis of such behaviour – 'boys will be boys' – indicating little hope for intervention or change.

Despite the distinction between 'natural' and 'social' here, both types of approach to social issues are examples of *social* construction. Each provides a way into defining, interpreting and acting in the social world that we inhabit. Each also provides a framework within which events, actions and types of people become meaningful, and which allows us to position ourselves in relation to them. However, the distinction between natural and social orientations is a significant one because of their different explanations of social behaviour. Different policy conclusions will also be drawn.

'Boys will be boys', but perhaps
in need of better role models?

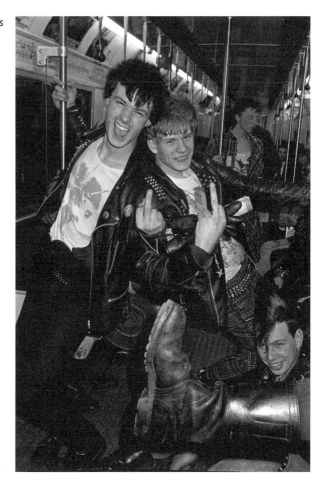

5.2 Levels of explanation

The distinction between the natural and the social is not the only significant
one. Even the social orientation in constructions of social problems is complicated
by different sorts of emphasis. The growth of social science since the late
nineteenth century has ensured that a variety of competing theories, disciplines
and perspectives are available to us in our attempt to make sense of social
problems. Such theories have made their way into the realm of everyday or
common-sense constructions – we all know bits of economic theory, bits of
psychology and even bits of sociology. For the purposes of this chapter, the
most useful way of distinguishing the differences in this approach involves
considering different *levels of explanation*.

Constructions that stress the 'social' conditions and causes of social issues
might begin with the level of the *individual*, looking at character, personality,
aptitudes, etc. Others might focus on the *family or kin group* of the individual –
how he or she is socialized, what behaviours, values, outlooks are learned or
acquired in the family setting. The third level would then be the *locality* – patterns
of social networks, peer groups and other local influences. Beyond this, one
might look to constructions that deal with the *culture* of a particular society – its
values, orientations and how these are communicated (the role of the mass

media, education system, and so on). Finally, some explanations look to *social structures* for the causes and conditions of problems – how the society is arranged, how the resources and power are distributed, and how inequality is organized. Different perspectives are likely to emphasize different levels of explanation.

ACTIVITY 1.5

Let us take another social issue, unemployment. Using the grid below, write against each level of explanation the factors you think would be important in constructing social explanations of unemployment.

Individual:
Familial:
Locality:
Cultural:
Structural:

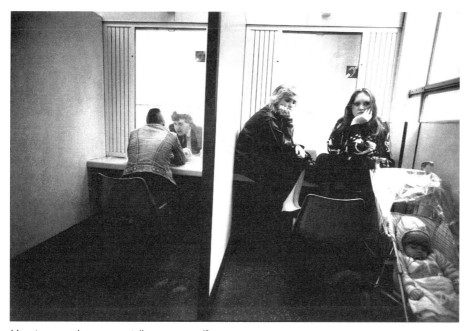

How is unemployment socially constructed?

We would have completed the grid as follows, but you may have had different answers.

Individual:	Explanations might address either the attitudes or capabilities of unemployed individuals. Are they actively looking for work, or are they work avoiders? Have they got the sorts of technical and social skills that employers are demanding?
Familial:	Has their upbringing or socialization prepared them adequately for the world of work? Have they got the right outlook? Are there family networks that help or hinder them in obtaining work?
Locality:	Are there particular possibilities or problems in the local pattern of employment? Are people part of a local culture which makes them less employable or less interested in work? Some people talk about local 'cultures of poverty' which pass on attitudes that make people less likely to look for or get jobs.
Cultural:	Do values in the wider society stress the merits of being employed? Do they promote responsibility? Or do they encourage dependency and idleness?
Structural:	Whose interests are served by unemployment? Does unemployment make labour cheaper or more manageable for employers? Why does the level or scale of unemployment change in different periods?

■ ■ ■

We do not intend this to be an exhaustive survey of all the different types of social explanations of unemployment, but we hope it illustrates the range and the way in which different levels provide a focus for such social explanations. A similar exercise could be undertaken for 'natural' constructions of unemployment and its causes. Are some people 'naturally' lazy or resistant to work? Is 'human nature' itself pleasure-seeking and work-avoiding? Do some people fail to respond to the sticks and carrots needed to make people work?

Summary

In this section we have tried to sketch some of the main lines of division in social constructions of social issues. The distinction between the natural and the social in constructing the causes that underlie social issues is a profound and recurrent one. A 'social' orientation involves the construction of social causes and conditions as the explanations for social issues. However, it is also important to bear in mind that such an orientation will itself be complicated by differences of perspective, particularly about the level of society upon which the construction focuses.

6   Scepticism and social construction

6.1   Common sense revisited

It is worth taking a little time to reflect on what we have discovered so far. Starting from 'what everybody knows' about a social problem – or what are sometimes called the *common-sense understandings* – allows us to see a number of things if we apply the scepticism of being a stranger in our own society.

First, there is a question about whether particular issues are commonly understood to be social problems. As we have seen, there are views which say either that poverty does not exist in the UK today, or that, if it does, it is not a social problem but a natural consequence of having a competitive society.

Second, we can see that common-sense understandings are not cut from a single cloth. In the case of poverty, we have seen that there are different views of poverty and its causes which pull in different directions. We can see these both in the form of simple statements and in the more developed form of arguments about poverty. This suggests that there is no absolute or clear-cut distinction between everyday or common-sense talk about poverty and academic analyses and arguments – a point to which we will return later in this chapter.

Third, we have seen that these multiple perspectives are not only different but that they are *contested*. That is to say, they aim to establish themselves as the 'correct' explanation, superior to others. These different perspectives are engaged in conflict about how to define and explain poverty. We can therefore suggest that the social construction of social problems is a contested process.

Fourth, each of the brief quotations in section 4 announces its claim to be the correct or true understanding of poverty in different ways. Let us look back at how this was done. The quotation from George Gilder talks about how 'fundamental realities' are concealed from the poor. Anderson talks about how some suggested solutions (that is, those from other perspectives) do not address the causes that he has identified. Oppenheim talks about low-paid and poorly protected employment being a 'hidden factor' which is revealed by her arguments. Each of them tells us about why they are superior perspectives. We can therefore suggest that particular social constructions of social problems attempt to establish themselves as 'true'.

The practice of systematic scepticism is an essential feature of social science in that it refuses to accept any of these self-proclaimed 'truths'. Each of them becomes something to be studied as part of the process by which social problems are socially constructed. It is one of the most challenging aspects of studying social science, since it demands that we distance ourselves not just from 'what everybody knows' but also from what we ourselves 'know' about social issues. 'What we know' is also part of the 'stock of knowledge' in this society. It is disconcerting to take the position of being a stranger, but it is necessary if we are to understand how social problems are socially constructed.

6.2   From social construction to social constructionism

social
constructionism

labelling

natural/
unnatural

The notion of social construction, we have argued, is fundamental to a social science approach to the analysis of social problems. However, some authors have developed the notion further into a more focused perspective, which may be called social constructionism. This perspective starts by emphasizing one essential feature of human societies – the role of language. In human societies, action is preceded by understanding and intention. We intend our actions to have meaningful outcomes. Our actions convey messages to other members of society. Although, as we shall see, some aspects of the social constructionist perspective can be quite complicated, it starts from a relatively simple point of departure. We might call this the naming or labelling of things. How we name things affects how we behave towards them. The name, or label, carries with it expectations.

Let us consider the example of motherhood. The link between the biological facts of motherhood and its social expression are frequently taken for granted. The social constructionist approach has a rather different starting point. Thus we expect mothers (or, more accurately, 'people who carry the label mother') to love their children, be attentive to their well-being and to enable them to thrive. The label 'mother' carries a stock of social expectations, so that if a mother fails to behave in this fashion – if she abandons or abuses her children – we are likely to identify her as 'unnatural' and will anticipate finding something wrong with her that would explain her failure to live up to our expectations. What matters here, say social constructionists, is not the biology but social expectations. As with the label 'mother', many other names (the socially constructed identities or patterns of our society) are so well established, or 'taken for granted', that we view them as natural. From a social constructionist standpoint, the appearance of the word natural (or unnatural) is usually a warning that deeply embedded patterns of social expectations are at stake. The most deeply embedded aspects of our social arrangements have become so 'taken for granted' that we find it hard to think of them as social. Instead, we attribute them to causes or forces beyond society – to the realm of nature.

The point here is not to deny that there are important biological or natural differences between people, or even to deny the existence of certain shared biological drives – as 'everybody knows', for example, we all have to eat. Rather, it is positively to affirm the importance of the ways in which such differences are given meaning through processes of social construction. Thus, the person who gives birth to a child is called a mother (although, of course, it is also possible to become a mother through adoption). However, it is not clear that the same assumptions are made about the behaviour that follows from this biological relationship in all societies, at all times, or in all classes. In contrast to the model outlined above, for example, in some societies infanticide has been an acceptable form of birth control; in others child care has been shared through wide kinship networks; and in some social classes and at some times the passing on of babies to wet-nurses and then nannies, with little continuing maternal contact, has been viewed positively. Licensed forms of abandonment might also include the sending of children to boarding school at an early age. In all of these contexts it is the social expectations rather than the biological necessity that matters. In broader terms, as is pointed out in Chapter 3, what matters is the various ways in which a bundle of 'natural material called the body is given a social meaning'.

Which are the 'natural' forms of child care?

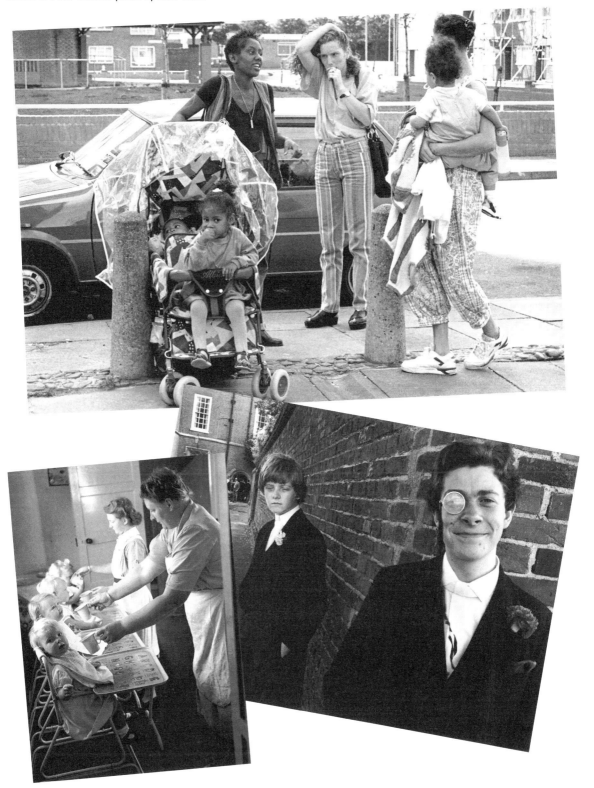

essentialism

Those who take a social constructionist approach (for example Burr, 1995) frequently contrast their position with what they characterize as essentialism Essentialism is the belief that social behaviour is determined by some underlying process or 'essence' which works itself out in social contexts. In this context it should not be confused with the more common everyday use of the word, in which 'essential' is defined as something one cannot do without. Most obviously, perhaps, essentialism finds a reflection in the notion that each of us has some basic personality which then determines the way in which we relate to others and fit into the wider social system. Similarly, the notion of some shared human nature can be seen as essentialist. Any argument which explains social or human behaviour largely in terms of biological functions or evolutionary pressures (for instance in terms of 'the survival of the fittest') can be seen as essentialist. Critics of essentialism have not, however, restricted themselves to questioning biological determinism: they question any explanation which suggests that the best way of understanding social phenomena is to analyse them to find some underlying truth just waiting to be exposed. So, for example, classical Marxism has been criticized because it sees history as the working out of fundamental conflicts between classes which are rooted within a capitalist mode of production.

ACTIVITY 1.6

Can you think of any other features of contemporary social arrangements that are represented as 'natural' or non-social? Jot down any you can think of. List also any social arrangements in which people do not act in line with conventional expectations and which are identified as 'unnatural'.

COMMENT

We are not going to try to write out our own list here, but instead we are going to suggest that most of the things that we define as 'natural' are areas of life where particular sorts of physical or biological features of human life are visible. For example, our expectations about how people of different ages should behave are often seen as natural (particularly with regard to the young and old). As a consequence, we may think of older people who do not behave in a dignified and restrained manner (as befits their age) as behaving unnaturally. Similarly, issues about differences between men and women, or regarding sexuality, are usually assigned to the 'natural' realm. We could give further examples, but the main point here is the way in which ideas about the 'natural' order of things usually conceal issues relating to social arrangements and our conventional expectations about them.

■ ■ ■

Social constructionism – as a way of studying social arrangements – starts from the rather mundane point that the naming of things affects how we act, and develops into an approach which sees the whole edifice of society as socially constructed. One of the earliest attempts to develop this approach, by the sociologists Peter Berger and Thomas Luckmann (1967), treated it as the means by which humans could create order out of the potential chaos of life. For them, social constructions simplified the business of living by establishing patterns of mutual expectations: mothers are like this, fathers are like this, children are like that, and so on. Such simplifying constructions were a form of energy-saving device. Rather than having to negotiate every aspect of life in each and every

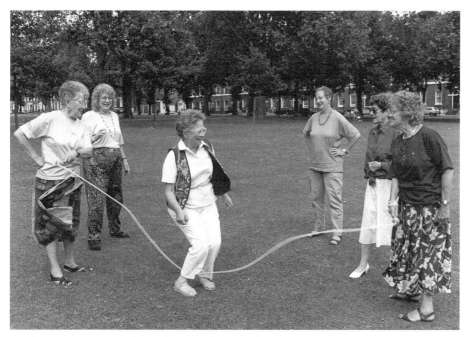

Defying our expectations of how older people should behave?

social encounter, social constructions – these simplifying typifications of people and behaviours – enabled people to proceed 'as if' we could all take these assumptions for granted. In time, such assumptions became habitualized – habits of mind that required little thought or attention. People forgot that they were constructions and they became naturalized – simply features of how the world is. In the process, people reproduced these constructions (and the assumptions behind them) in their behaviour. The social order is produced and reproduced through the ways in which we enact these social constructions. As individuals we find ourselves operating within a limited range of choice of positions – sometimes called subject positions – within that social order. For example, a mother may find herself exploring the options of housewife, working mother or single mother, each of which is constructed as a set of expectations about how she will act.

subject positions

Berger and Luckmann's view of social construction is only one strand in the development of this perspective (see Burr, 1995, for a fuller introduction to social constructionism). In the following sections we will be looking at the possible links between the social constructionist approach and concepts of 'ideology' and 'discourse'. However, what all of the different strands that have contributed to the perspective have in common is their stress on the way in which collective or shared understandings, interpretations or representations of the world shape our actions within it. Where they differ is in how they view these constructions. Some, particularly those associated with the concept of ideology, see constructions as a means through which social groups promote or legitimate their interests. Others, more closely associated with the idea of discourse, see social constructions as forming, rather than reflecting, social identities and interests.

Summary

Common sense is a complex and contested phenomenon. The practice of systematic scepticism is a key aspect of social science, particularly in the analysis of common sense and the consideration of the social construction of social problems. Social constructionism emphasizes the importance of social expectations in the analysis of taken-for-granted and apparently natural social processes. It starts by exploring the assumptions associated with the naming or labelling of things. It is sceptical about any form of essentialism, which seeks to explain social phenomena in terms of natural or biological drives.

7   The question of ideology: social interests and social constructions

7.1   Legitimating the powerful

The labelling perspective associated with Berger and Luckmann focuses on the processes by which some behaviours and types of people become marked out for social disapproval – targeted by the wider society as different and requiring some form of social response. Its virtue is that it challenges conventional assumptions that social problems exist 'out there' as obvious and commonly understood facts. Berger and Luckmann's perspective stresses the importance of language in shaping how we define, understand and respond to social problems by drawing attention to the role of labelling. However, the perspective is less helpful in dealing with the question of why some conditions become identified as problems and why some sorts of social constructions are in widespread use. One of the ways in which the labelling perspective has been developed is through linking social construction to issues of social interests, power and ideologies.

In this view, societies are characterized by patterns of inequality between social groups, for instance between different classes, between men and women, or between different ethnic groups. Groups in dominant positions in society will try to use sets of ideas that legitimate existing arrangements – and their positions within them. For example, groups or classes who control a large share of a society's wealth are likely to spread ideas about the necessity or even desirability of these patterns of economic inequality. They may refer to the fact that wealth reflects social virtue ('breeding') or accomplishment (the reward for 'risk-taking'). They may argue that inequality is necessary to encourage everyone to strive to be successful. They may argue that wealth is a responsibility held in trust for future generations. Such sets of ideas that legitimate advantageous

ideology

positions tend to be called ideologies. Similar ideologies have been used to justify the inequalities between men and women (men are stronger, better at thinking abstractly; women are better at caring or need to conserve their resources for the demands of childbirth, and so on). As both these examples suggest, one common feature of such ideologies is that they claim that existing social arrangements are legitimate because they are 'natural' (and therefore both desirable and unavoidable). Each structural pattern of inequality is likely to create interests (in preserving or changing the existing pattern) and these interests are likely to provide the foundation for ideologies which seek to legitimate or challenge these inequalities.

This is the most simple view of ideology: as a set of ideas which attempt to legitimate (or challenge) social position and inequality. Even in this most simple form, however, we can see ways in which it can link to and develop the labelling approach to social construction.

Let us return to the issue of poverty. How might poverty be defined in ways which would reinforce or challenge the position of the powerful?

COMMENT

We suggest that it might be in the interests of those with wealth to deny that poverty is a social problem (or even that it exists). If poverty can be explained as being the result of 'sad, bad or mad' people – those who are workshy, feckless or incompetent – then poverty is nothing to do with the social arrangements that make some people wealthy. Alternatively, poverty can be explained as a necessary, if unfortunate, by-product of a system that creates wealth. We might even go so far as to say that the idea of poverty is itself tolerable within such an ideology because it separates out the 'poor' as a social problem, rather than revealing the underlying structure of inequality. In distinguishing between the normal and the deviant, the wider inequalities and differences of social interest are concealed. On the other hand, if poverty were solely blamed either on the behaviour of the rich or on the operation of an unfair or unjust economic system, it might underpin a political ideology which aimed to challenge the powerful in society.

■ ■ ■

Ideologies are also likely to be involved in defining who and what are social problems. Most obviously, those who challenge existing social arrangements are likely to be defined as troublemakers, agitators or rabble-rousers who aim to cause unnecessary social disruption and disaffection. Alternatively, such challenges may be dismissed as utopian, unworldly or even unnatural because they claim that other ways of arranging the social world are possible. Beyond this, however, there are ways in which specific social conditions or patterns of behaviour might be identified as social problems because they run counter to the interests of dominant groups. For example, some social scientists have suggested that the interests of a capitalist class mean that it needs a healthy and reliable workforce. In the period of industrialization, therefore, indolence and insobriety came to be defined as social problems because they threatened to disrupt patterns of work and the norm of a sober and industrious worker (see, for example, Clarke and Critcher, 1985). Equally, it has been argued that the industrialists of Britain came to take a growing interest in the 'health of the nation' at the end of the nineteenth century, when they became concerned that ill-health and malnutrition made the British working class less fit and less competitive by comparison with other industrializing nations. Social problems here are the result of interests being threatened, and the definitions of those problems stem from the power of dominant groups to determine what counts as a problem.

In this view ideologies are *functional.* That is, they are geared to legitimating social positions. In principle, one can look behind ideologies to see what interests they protect and serve. They are also intended to *mystify* or *conceal* what society is really like by explaining away inequalities. So, for example, these legitimating ideologies may celebrate forms of equality (equality before the law, for instance) which distract attention from other areas of social life where inequality is rife. Anatole France referred ironically to 'the majestic equality of the French law, which forbids both rich and poor from sleeping under the bridges of the Seine' (quoted in CSE/NDC, 1977, pp.24–5).

7.2   Contesting ideologies

Much social science analysis has been devoted to exploring the variants and consequences of this simple view of ideology, including capitalist ideology, which legitimates the interests of owners of capital against the working class; patriarchal ideology, which legitimates the interests of men against women; and racist ideology, which legitimates the interests of dominant ethnic groups against others – most evidently in the ideology of apartheid in South Africa. However, this simple and functionalist conception of ideology has been developed in a number of ways. First, as we have already hinted, the stress on 'dominant' ideologies which legitimate social interests has been tempered by a recognition that there are other ideologies which challenge and contest dominant ones. For example, one might consider the conflicts between capitalist and socialist ideologies which sought to challenge or change the structural inequalities of capitalist societies; the conflicts between patriarchal and feminist ideologies over gender inequalities; or those between racist and anti-racist ideologies around inequalities of 'race' and ethnicity. Opening up ideologies in this way gives a more *dynamic* view of ideological conflict and struggles.

Oppositional ideologies are likely to try to define different sorts of social problems. Thus, socialist ideologies define inequality and its effects as social problems; feminist ideologies define gender differences in income, work and access to power (as well as issues of male violence within and outside home) as social problems; and anti-racist ideologies have attempted to construct inequalities (of income and rights) and other dimensions of racism (such as vulnerability to racially motivated attacks) as social problems. In this sense, one can treat the public agenda of social problems as one focus of ideological conflict in which competing ideologies struggle to establish their definitions of social problems, and what needs to be done about them.

ACTIVITY 1.8

Age is another issue around which there are contested understandings. Some would suggest that no one other than a mature adult is capable of taking full control of his or her own life. Consider, first, what might be the dominant ideologies behind this statement. Whose social interests do you think would be legitimated by it? Then try to identify alternative or counter-ideologies and the social interests which might underlie them. Finally, think about some of the contradictory common-sense views that surround the notion of growing old.

In generational terms the statement clearly supports the position of mature adults – that is, those who already tend to be in more powerful positions at home and at work. It might therefore also be seen as a statement which underpins structures of social order and minimizes the risk of challenge from below – young people have to learn and accept discipline. It may also imply that those who have moved into old age need to accept secondary status. It is consistent with the view that those outside the workforce are a drain on the resources of those who are in productive employment.

Powerful counter-ideologies are also available, of course. From the young it might be argued that many people are already over the hill at 30, in some occupations at least. It might also be claimed that the young alone represent the hope of the future. Older people might emphasize the value of experience and wisdom, as well as stressing their entitlement to some support after a lifetime of supporting others. Each of these arguments would be appealing to different 'bits' of common sense.

■ ■ ■

One approach to the concept of ideology links it to the issue of common sense, which we discussed earlier. This approach derives from the work of the Italian Marxist Antonio Gramsci (1971; see also Hall, Lumley and McLennan, 1978) and is concerned with the way in which conflicting ideologies contend over common-sense understandings. In this approach, ideologies struggle to establish their legitimacy and power by drawing connections with aspects of everyday or common-sense knowledge. In doing so, they try to organize and mobilize elements of common-sense knowledge as part of their world view and in support of the social interests they represent. Thus, dominant social classes will refer to, and make connections with, aspects of common-sense knowledge that reflect and support existing patterns of inequality and which legitimate the economic or political power of these dominant groups. Counter-ideologies will want to build connections with those other elements of common-sense thought that object to or are sceptical about the existing social order.

In this perspective, common sense – understood as the contradictory and complex package of 'bits' discussed earlier – forms a field that is selectively addressed by contending ideologies. Different ideologies will address different 'bits' and try to organize them into a coherent story and a particular sort of perspective on the world. The aim is to ensure that there appears to be no alternative to the vision of society being presented that is capable of winning tacit or active support from people across a wide social spectrum. Gramsci used the term hegemonic to describe a political project that achieved these ends. **hegemonic**

A particular example of this was provided in the 1980s by the ideology of the New Right associated with the Thatcher government in Britain and the Reagan **New Right**
presidency in the USA. This ideology was committed to social and economic programmes that would create an increased role for market forces and a more dynamic – if more unequal – capitalism, and was addressed to those aspects of common sense which saw competition, inequality and individualism as the dominant, and desirable, characteristics of social and economic life (Levitas, 1986; Hall, 1988). Thus New Right ideology addressed the 'natural' state of economic competition, identifying it as an essential feature of life for individuals, companies and even nations ('Great Britain plc') (these issues are discussed

further in **Hughes and Lewis, 1998**). It stressed those parts of common sense that focused on individual freedoms (to earn and spend money) rather than collective provision (the 'nanny state' supported by 'excessive taxation'). Although this ideology often presented itself as common sense, it is important to recognize that it addressed common-sense thought *selectively*. It ignored or repressed those 'bits' of common sense that did not fit or could not be integrated into this ideological direction – in particular, those 'bits' that supported collective provision, mutual dependency, intergenerational solidarity, and so forth. Such 'bits' were usually demonized as 'socialism'.

This brief sketch, simplifying a complex process of ideological work, is intended to indicate that the relationship between ideologies and common sense may be a central issue in how social issues and social problems are constructed.

Summary

Taking the question of ideology seriously provides a way of developing beyond the limitations of the labelling perspective in studying the social construction of social problems in three main ways:

1   Foregrounding ideology allows us to ask the questions: who says this is a social problem, and whose interests are being served by this definition? Looking at ideologies reminds us that the ways in which problems are identified and defined are neither obvious nor neutral but are *socially motivated*.

2   The issue of ideology also directs attention to *what sorts of solutions* are being proposed or are implied in the way the problem is constructed. These too are socially motivated.

3   The idea of *conflicting ideologies* provides a reminder that there is usually more than one definition of social problems in play – both in the definition of what conditions are social problems, and about how any particular problem should be defined and understood.

8   Norms, truth and power: discourses of social problems

8.1   Ideologies and discourses

Some social scientists, following the French writer Michel Foucault (1972, 1976, 1979), have argued that the view of ideology developed in section 7 is too narrow because of the link that it creates between sets of ideas and the interests of specific social groups – for example, in identifying a capitalist ideology as if ideas go around with number plates on their back which allow us to see whose ideas they are. They suggest that we need a more complex view of how social knowledges are organized and distributed and of their consequences for social action. Foucault used the term discourses rather than ideologies. He studied how knowledges about a range of social issues emerged and shaped patterns of social action, including such focal points as madness, the prison system and

discourse

sexuality. The idea of discourses is an important one for studying the social construction of social problems. It draws on the everyday meaning of the word discourse – to 'talk about' – to emphasize that knowledges are carried and reproduced through 'talk' and 'writing'. Societies 'discourse about' their social problems and social policies in a variety of ways – in political statements, television programmes, social science studies and 'everyday' conversations.

Foucault's view of discourses takes a step further, however. He suggests that each discourse is structured or organized around central themes and connections, and these define the terms in which statements can be made, investigations conducted, and conversations can take place. For example, in talking about 'poverty' we are already within a discourse that shapes what can be said. Let us look at some of these organizing principles of the discourse on poverty and their consequences:

- To talk about poverty is to take a view of inequality as a difference between two positions. The population can be divided into the 'non-poor' and the 'poor'. There are other views of inequality (other discourses) that do not take this view, but which see it as a more complex structure, either with different layers or as a relational process.

- The distinction between the non-poor and the poor means that attention is concentrated on the poor: they are the deviations from the norm of being not-poor. This discourse therefore means that arguments will centre on how to define the poor, how many poor people there are, whether numbers have risen or fallen, and how to explain their condition. Although there may be different theories of poverty, they contend and offer their competing explanations within the discourse of poverty.

- The concentration on the poor in the discourse of poverty means that attention and explanations tend to centre on 'what makes them poor', and this usually means looking for what it is about them (their attitudes, character, behaviour) that makes them (rather than us) become or remain poor.

- As a result, the 'poor' become the subject of investigations, inquiries and studies designed to examine them and their 'forms of life' (Dean, 1991). The discourse of poverty means that we know far more about how the poor live than any other social group. We know about their housing, their spending patterns, their dietary habits, the ways in which they raise children, how they spend their days, their health patterns and even how they die and are buried (the pauper's grave). The discourse of poverty organizes social knowledge in particular ways: 'we' (the rest of society) look *at* poor people.

8.2   The institutionalization of discourses

We can see discourses as ways of organizing knowledge. They define what the problem is; they say what is worth knowing and what can be said. They produce the 'norms' against which deviation or abnormality is marked (the norm of 'not being poor', for example). But discourses are not just about words. Discourses shape and become institutionalized in social policies and the organizations through which they are carried out. This is not just a matter of the big policy ideas – the pressure to 'do something about poverty' – but also the minute arrangements by which 'something is done'. Let us give some more examples about poverty and how the discourse of poverty has been institutionalized.

- *Poor people have to prove that they are poor.* The systems of doing something about poverty – what in the nineteenth century used to be called providing 'poor relief' – have always involved various sorts of tests that poor people have to pass to prove their need. For example, there have been availability for work tests, in which the poor must prove that they are ready to help themselves by taking work if it is available. There have been means tests, assessing household income to see that it falls below the agreed line at which benefits will be paid. There have also been morality tests – mainly directed at women – which examine whether they are cohabiting and thus potentially dependent on a man's income.

- *Poor people must present themselves as poor.* They are 'claimants' – an inferior and dependent social status, asking for something from society. Many social benefits go unclaimed, partly for reasons of access to information about them, but also partly because of the stigma (the social taint) of being a claimant. Once people place themselves within the discourse of poverty, their identity is defined in its terms. They are positioned as 'subjects' within it – that is, they are themselves subjects of the discourse and understand their own position through it.

- *Poor people have things* done to *them*. Being poor is to be placed in a position where other people have rights over you. Society's institutional arrangements have sometimes focused on *segregating* the poor – putting them in workhouses, for example – to keep them away from the rest of 'us'. Sometimes they have been concerned to *normalize* the poor – giving lessons in budgetary management, good housekeeping, or parenting – with the aim of making 'them' more like 'us'. At other times the emphasis has been on maintaining *surveillance* on the poor – monitoring their behaviour to make sure that they behave 'properly'. Although different policies on poverty aim to do different things, they are framed by the discourse of poverty in that they see poor people as the objects of policy – people to whom things are done (often 'in their own best interests').

power

Discourses in this sense are also about relations of power. They organize positions and places in a field of power. So, in relation to poverty, they empower (give power to) state agencies to monitor, assess or intervene in the lives of poor people. They empower some agencies (both state and voluntary agencies) to evaluate the 'worth' or 'desert' of poor people before benefits or services are provided. Discourses may also – conditionally – empower or give power to poor people. Poor people may be 'enabled' to look for work, to take courses, to

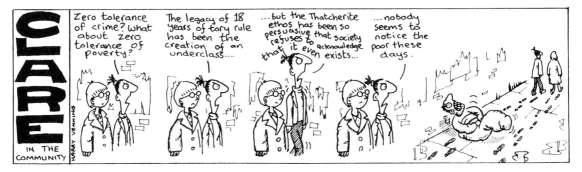

receive extra benefits, to keep their children, so long as they prove that they are the 'right sort' of poor people.

Extract 1.1 is a document produced by the Charity Organization Society, a nineteenth-century voluntary organization which offered 'relief' to poor people who met its criteria. What view of poverty and poor people does it represent?

Extract 1.1 Charity Organization Society: 'Notice to persons applying for assistance'

1   The Society desires to help those persons who are doing all they can to help themselves, and to whom temporary assistance is likely to prove a lasting benefit.

2   No assistance should be looked for without full information being given in order that the Committee may be able to judge:

    (a) Whether the applicant ought to be helped by charity.

    (b) What is the best way of helping them …

3   Persons wishing to be assisted by loans must find satisfactory security, such as that of respectable householders … Loans must be paid back by regular instalments.

4   Persons who have thrown themselves out of employment through their own fault ought not to count on being helped by charity.

5   Persons of drunken, immoral or idle habits can not expect to be assisted unless they can satisfy the Committee that they are really trying to reform.

6   The Society does not, unless under exceptional circumstances, give or obtain help for the payment of back rent or funeral expenses. But when help of this sort is asked for, there may be other and better ways of assisting.

7   Assistance will not, as a rule, be given in addition to a Parish allowance.

By Order,
COS Committee

COMMENT

The emphasis of the COS regulations is relatively clear, making a fundamental distinction between the deserving and undeserving poor. Help will be given to those who 'are doing all they can to help themselves'. Those who have 'drunken, immoral or idle habits' will not receive assistance. In other words, the emphasis is overwhelmingly placed on the individual characteristics of poor people, and assistance is provided only to those who can be helped out of temporary difficulties, where 'temporary assistance is likely to prove a lasting benefit'. Within the discourse of the COS, it is not possible to view poverty as an endemic feature of society, a consequence of social and economic structures which foster inequality. Poor people become positioned as supplicants, whose own behaviour explains their poverty.

■ ■ ■

Summary

The idea of discourse alerts us to a number of issues about the social construction of social problems. It suggests that we need to look beyond competing theories or perspectives to look at how knowledge is organized around central themes that allow the different theories to compete. Discourses define what the problem is, and it is because theories share the definition of the problem that they can compete and argue. Perspectives that start somewhere else – or do not share the definition of the problem – have great difficulty in making themselves heard or understood. They do not fit the terms of reference of the discourse. Thus the discourse represented by the COS rules is not one that would allow for the discussion of poverty either as a consequence of the behaviour of the rich or as a consequence of structural social inequalities.

Second, discourses shape what sorts of knowledge are meaningful, worth having and 'truthful'. As we have seen, the discourse of poverty means that we look for, collect and use knowledge about 'poor people'. To suggest that this category of people does not exist, or that we should not try to know more about them sounds *meaningless*. Of course, 'everybody knows' that there are poor people. They can be identified, measured and investigated (and we can only do something about the problem of poverty if we know more about it). But the *category* of 'poor people' only exists because of the discourse of poverty, and we should not assume that 'they' are 'different' because of that. Placing 'them' in a separate category can be seen as a means of marginalizing or excluding 'them' from normal life.

Third, the idea of discourse points us to the importance of looking at the ways in which the poor are institutionalized in social arrangements and relations of power. The workhouse, charity organizations, benefits offices, means tests, cohabitation rules and so on are ways in which the discourse of poverty has been institutionalized (and they also reflect different sorts of theories, policies and perspectives within the discourse). They involve relations of power between groups of social actors – claimants, assessors, case workers, fraud investigators, and so on. The next chapter develops some of these points in greater depth, with a specific focus on the medical discourse on disability.

9   Conclusion: the view from social constructionism

This chapter has concentrated on the question of how social issues are socially constructed. It has done so not because this is the only form of analysis in the social sciences. There are many different approaches, theories and perspectives that bear upon social problems, patterns of social differentiation and the organization of social welfare. Nevertheless, all of them have to operate in a social world where *the meaning of things* shapes how we act. It is this that makes processes of social construction such a central focus for the study of social issues. As we have seen, there are different ways of engaging with studying social constructions – we can treat them as labels, forms of knowledge, ideologies or discourses – but it is difficult to proceed without studying them. However, it is important to end this chapter with two cautionary points. The first concerns the fragility of social constructions. The second concerns the relationship between social constructionism and politics.

The focus on social construction often sounds rather ethereal, dealing with fragile tissues of what things mean and how they are interpreted or defined. This all sounds rather intangible alongside what is often referred to as the 'real world' – hard facts, solid structures and grim realities. Indeed, part of the attraction of social constructionism as a perspective is that it suggests the social world might be slightly less solid and permanent than such emphasis on the 'hard facts of life' might imply. Social constructionism does, after all, indicate that the social world is constructed – meanings are made, definitions produced and interpretations propounded. In this way, social constructionism highlights the *provisional* character of social life: in other words, what was constructed this way could have been constructed differently. It implies a degree of fragility or impermanence in social arrangements. Social constructionism, as a way of looking at the world, implies the possibility of other constructions.

Nevertheless, it would be a mistake to confuse social constructionism as a perspective – the way of looking – with the lives of particular social constructions. The perspective may imply impermanence or fragility: the idea that the social world is fluid or changeable. But this is not the same as saying that all social constructions are fluid, changeable or intangible. Nor does it mean that they do not have real consequences for people as they live their lives. Many social constructions are deeply embedded or solidified as ways of thinking and acting that change hardly at all. Despite the impact of competing constructions like feminism, many of our social constructions about men and women have resisted change. They remain deeply rooted in 'natural' orientations about what men and women are 'really' like. As a consequence, we encounter the sorts of contradictory common sense that we saw earlier in relation to poverty. As regards gender, though, 'what everybody knows' might include the knowledge that: there is a 'glass ceiling' that stops women being promoted; men are better managers; equal opportunities have gone too far; men can't get a fair deal; women who want careers are unnatural; and men should have the same rights as women to look after children. Confusing and contradictory this array may be, but it is the product of overlaid forms of competing constructions – some long-standing and deeply sedimented in our society but intersecting with others which challenge and attempt to change the ways we think and act.

In this respect, social constructions should not be seen as fragile, insubstantial or impermanent. Berger and Luckmann (1967, pp.65–89) discuss three interlinked processes through which social constructions become solidified: *habitualization, institutionalization* and *sedimentation*. Each of these processes relates to the way human societies build patterns of predictability and stability that are reproduced over time. The reproduction of social arrangements requires predictability – the development of habits of thought and action that impose a social order. Berger and Luckmann argue that:

> All human activity is subject to habitualization. Any action that is repeated frequently becomes cast into a pattern, which can then be reproduced with an economy of effort … Habitualization further implies that the action in question may be performed again and again in the same manner and with the same economic effort.
>
> (Berger and Luckmann, 1967, p.71)

The fact that this order is socially constructed does not make it any less real.

Berger and Luckmann deal with the way in which social constructions become institutionalized as the 'taken for granted' facts of everyday life. Although these 'habits' may be socially constructed, each individual encounters them as social facts – they are solidified and intransigent. We face these as institutions to which *we* have to adjust. What the perspective of social construction allows us to see is the way in which a social order – its habits, institutions, characteristic ways of thinking and acting – is both socially produced and appears as the natural and proper way of behaving. Over time, patterns of human behaviour are laid down, or sedimented, and each new development has to relate to the sediments of the past. The social constructionist perspective enables us to understand both stability (the reproduction of this social order) and change, as competing constructions attempt to break old habits and create new ones. The perspective of social constructionism allows us to see these social arrangements as both fragile and solid, permanent and changeable. So, when we explore the social construction of social problems, we can see how particular ways of thinking and acting become 'habits', institutionalized and 'sedimented' as the normal way of life.

To many people, it has appeared that social constructionism is equivalent to a radical political stance. To point out the constructed nature of social arrangements does raise challenging issues. Indeed, some social and political movements have used the perspective of social constructionism to argue for the need to change existing or dominant constructions. For example, some versions of feminism developed challenges to dominant images, expectations and constructions of femininity as oppressive, exploitative and legitimating forms of inequality. However, social constructionism as a perspective is not equivalent to any particular form of politics. As a perspective, it is politically agnostic – it makes no direct political claims of its own – except about claims that the social order is natural, eternal, immutable or otherwise fixed. Social constructionism presents an inherent challenge to such claims because of the insistence on social orders being socially constructed. But beyond that, social constructionism has no intrinsic politics. It leaves open the question of what sort of social constructions would be most desirable. These are the focus of political choice, conflict and argument.

Such matters cannot be resolved by or within a social constructionist perspective. It may be that, like most social science, social constructionism is 'inherently disturbing or critical, because to look for explanations of what is normally taken for granted as natural … runs counter to the norms of everyday behaviour' (Platt, 1991, p.345). In that sense, the practice of scepticism, the taking up of the role of a 'stranger' in one's own society, and the insistence that social orders are socially constructed, is disconcerting. It involves a perspective which refuses to 'take for granted'. But it is a perspective, not a politics. Social constructionism is, above all, a method of analysing social arrangements. What to do about them is a question that follows from the analysis: the method does not presuppose any particular conclusion.

The later chapters of this book utilize social constructionism to explore a range of social issues or social 'problems'. The topics explored are of vital importance in themselves, but each chapter also illustrates the value of social constructionism as a method. Together they show how the social constructionist perspective can be used effectively in the analysis of contemporary social policy. Chapter 2 focuses on social constructions of disability, and particularly on the ways in which disability has been medicalized – viewed through the social construction given by the medical perspective. In Chapter 3 the focus of attention shifts to the social construction of 'race' and ethnicity, specifically considering the way in which discourses of 'race' have operated in the field of education policy. It shows the power of such discourses in shaping the lived experience of children and parents in the education system. Chapter 4 turns to issues of sexuality, specifically the social construction of 'deviant' sexualities, and the emergence of 'the homosexual', as well as considering the ways in which prostitution has been defined and redefined since the nineteenth century. Chapter 5 concludes the book. It revisits the themes of the book, highlighting the ways in which the social constructionist perspective has been used in earlier chapters.

At the centre of all the chapters is an attempt to explore the ways in which social differences are constructed. The issues explored in the various chapters are sensitive and challenging ones. They may sometimes raise points that make you uneasy or challenge deeply-held convictions about the way the world works and your position in it. We believe, however, that it is only by approaching issues systematically with the help of a social constructionist perspective that the emergence of social problems and the development of social policy can be explored effectively.

Further reading

Berger and Luckmann (1967) is a classic text in the development of the social constructionist perspective within the sociological tradition. Burr (1995) offers a very thorough review of the social constructionist perspective, clearly outlining the methods of discourse analysis. Although the book draws significantly on debates within social psychology, it is of wide relevance to the social sciences more generally.

References

Anderson, D. (1991) *The Unmentionable Face of Poverty in the Nineties: Domestic Incompetence, Improvidence and Male Irresponsibility in Low Income Families*, London, Social Affairs Unit.

Barash, P. (1981) *Sociobiology: The Whisperings Within*, London, Fontana.

Berger, P. and Luckmann, T. (1967) *The Social Construction of Reality*, London, Allen Lane.

Burr, V. (1995) *An Introduction to Social Constructionism*, London, Routledge.

Clarke, J. and Critcher, C. (1985) *The Devil Makes Work: Leisure in Capitalist Britain*, London, Macmillan.

CSE/NDC (eds) (1977) *Capitalism and the Rule of Law*, London, Macmillan on behalf of Conference of Socialist Economists/National Deviancy Conference.

Dean, M. (1991) *The Constitution of Poverty*, London, Routledge.

Foucault, M. (1972) *The Archaeology of Knowledge*, London, Tavistock.

Foucault, M. (1976) *The History of Sexuality. An Introduction*, Harmondsworth, Penguin.

Foucault, M. (1979) *Discipline and Punish*, Harmondsworth, Penguin.

Gilder, G. (1981) *Wealth and Poverty*, New York, Basic Books.

Gramsci, A. (1971) *Selections from the Prison Notebooks*, London, Lawrence and Wishart.

Hall, S. (1988) *The Hard Road to Renewal*, London, Verso.

Hall, S., Lumley, R. and McLennan, G. (1978) 'Politics and ideology: Gramsci', in Centre for Contemporary Cultural Studies, *On Ideology*, London, Hutchinson.

Herrnstein, R.T. and Murray, C. (1994) *The Bell Curve. Intelligence and Class Structure in American Life*, New York, Free Press.

Hughes, G. and Lewis, G. (1998) *Unsettling Welfare: The Reconstruction of Social Policy*, **London, Routledge in association with The Open University.**

Levitas, R. (ed.) (1986) *The Ideology of the New Right*, Cambridge, Polity Press.

Mills, C.W. (1959) *The Sociological Imagination*, Oxford, Oxford University Press.

Oppenheim, C. (1993) *Poverty: The Facts*, London, Child Poverty Action Group.

Platt, J. (1991) 'The contribution of social science', in Loney, M. *et al.* (eds) *The State or the Market: Politics and Welfare in Contemporary Britain*, second edition, London, Sage.

Wilson, G. (1981) *Love and Instinct*, London, Temple Smith.

CHAPTER 2

A Suitable Case for Treatment? Constructions of Disability

by Gordon Hughes

Contents

1   Introduction

The key aim of this chapter is to consolidate further your understanding of social constructionism as a method for examining how different groups of people and types of behaviour come to be viewed as social problems or social issues about which something needs to be done. The chapter examines both the construction of different categories of individuals and the organized interventions directed towards them, using the example of disability to illustrate the method of social constructionism. Thus we examine how disability is, was and will be the subject of different and conflicting constructions regarding its 'nature' and 'meaning'. However, it is vital to remember that such constructions and categorizations are not the exclusive preserve of those people, acts or behaviour that are identified as 'deviant' or 'social problems'. All social phenomena are subject to such constructing and deconstructing processes over time.

The chapter is structured as follows:

- Section 2 introduces you to some of the key contemporary representations of disabled people in the media, and asks: what are the dominant popular images and labels of disability, and has this imagery 'cast' disabled people in a particular way? This section also explores how dominant popular representations of disability may themselves be subject to contestation and thus deconstruction.

- Section 3 asks a series of questions about both the definition and measurement of disability, and presents a specific illustration of how social scientific analysis contributes to the study of social issues, in this case disability.

- Section 4 explores the historical roots of our contemporary common-sense notions of disability. In particular it examines the role and influence of religious and moralistic ideas in producing a construction of the disabled person as 'the other'. The discussion also focuses on how such a construction has been institutionalized in the discourse of 'disability charities'.

- Section 5 examines how a medical discourse became (and remains) the dominant expert construction of disability in the twentieth century. Particular attention is given to the ways in which a powerful knowledge (in this case 'scientific' medical knowledge) was able to take ownership of a problem and realize its power through specific institutionalized practices.

- Finally, section 6 explores the growth of an alternative framework for understanding disability to that of the medical discourse, namely the social model of disability. Attention is also paid to the contested nature of this social mode of analysis.

You should be aware that our concerns are chiefly about the uses of social constructionism as a social scientific method for understanding social phenomena. Remember that disability is used primarily as an illustrative example, so you should not expect this chapter to tell you the 'story' of disability.

2 Popular representations of disabled people

Disability has historically been a taboo subject. The varied experiences of disabled people have been hidden from history and have only recently become a subject for sustained and critical social scientific analysis. The relative hiddenness of disability as a social phenomenon is particularly striking when we compare coverage of disability issues in the media and in political debates with other social issues such as unemployment and crime.

When was the last time you saw, heard or read a news item on disabled people in the national media? Think carefully about this, and then consider the news coverage on criminals.

It is very unlikely that you will have come across much coverage of disability in the national newspapers, or on radio or television. As Barnes (1992) has shown, despite the campaigning by the disability movement in the last decades of the twentieth century in the UK and elsewhere, disability remains largely a taboo topic in the media, the exceptions being the tales of tragedy or heroism by exceptional individuals or the often dramatic representations in charity advertisements (of which more in section 4.2).

The claim that disability is a taboo topic in many social situations may need some further explanation. According to anthropologists, a taboo is a thing, person or act that is subject to social or sacred prohibition and thereby rendered untouchable or unmentionable. In your experience you may well have encountered such informal prohibitions on talking about disability. Furthermore, anthropologists have suggested that a major function performed by taboos may be as a subtle mechanism of social control. Thus the existence of taboos may make the world a more orderly and easily classified place by the establishment of clear boundary marks between 'normal' and 'abnormal', 'safe' and 'dangerous', 'natural' and 'unnatural', 'pure' and 'impure' (Douglas, 1966).

So far we have suggested that disability as a phenomenon remains largely hidden and for the most part untalked about in contemporary popular representations of the social world. However, images and stereotypes of disabled people, often negative but sometimes positive, are present to us all in often striking and disturbing ways.

representation

ACTIVITY 2.1

Study the representations of disabled people, both factual and fictional, in Extracts 2.1–2.5, and then think about the following questions:

1   With regard to Extracts 2.1 and 2.2, what major imagery of disabled people is conveyed in each news story? What are the common expressions used to describe the experiences of the two men featured in the articles?

2   What are the dominant and competing stereotypes of disability in the fictional depictions of disabled people in the children's literature in Extracts 2.3 and 2.4?

3   Compare these images with the list of assumptions and ideas identified in Extract 2.5 by Pam Evans, an activist in the disability movement, as being the essence of the day-to-day prejudice that disabled people face.

4   How might Extract 2.5 open up alternative ways of seeing disabled people beyond that of negative stereotyping?

The challenge facing you here is that of working with different sources of evidence. Try to think about the different devices, such as the use of certain key words and style of language, that are used in the different types of source material.

Extract 2.1 *Haringey Weekly Herald*: 'The best of British'

Phil fights deafness to lead chess challenge

Move over Gary Kasparov. It's time to check out Phillip Gardner who's on the way to becoming king of the chessboards against stiff East European competition.

For Phillip, of College Road, Tottenham, is a member of an extraordinary chess team which will be taking part in an international tournament this year.

The 32-year-old computer analyst and his four team-mates are fighting their way to the top with the odds stacked against them. They are all deaf.

(*Haringey Weekly Herald and North London Advertiser*, 10 January 1990)

Extract 2.2 *Star Sunday Sport*: '27 years of hell – and he's still smiling'

Heartless idiots laughed at his knobbly face … and webbed hands and feet.

Children drove him to tears with cruel taunts. And pretty girls broke his heart. But ugly duckling Andrew Dickson refused to hide away.

And now, after a staggering £2 million worth of hospital treatment, his smile says it all.

Andrew has suffered 27 years of torment – and 70 operations. His story is one of immense courage.

'I looked like Frankenstein when I was born … drooping forehead, webbed hands and feet, and a nose as flat as a snout.

My parents, Vera and Eric, were shattered. But they refused to hide me away like the legendary Victorian freak John Merrick.

I had my first operation when I was just five weeks old.

Great Ormond Street surgeons defied nature, slicing my hands, building a nose, and transplanting a rib to my forehead.

The National Health Service must have spent £2 million on me.

It was sheer hell. But I'll never regret it, even though I still have webbed feet.

When I was ten I was offered a life-or-death operation. It had only been tried once before and it was very risky. But it worked wonders. I began to hope that one day I might look normal.

I shake with pain at the memories of my teenage years.

I never used to go out in the evenings as I only had a couple of friends. Most kids made fun of me.

And I nearly cried when I saw the Elephant Man film, because that was what it was like for me. Children at school were so, so cruel.

I'm 27 now, but I still feel nervous if I go swimming at strange baths because I'm afraid people will stare.

But that's the only time I worry – except when it comes to girlfriends.

I've only asked two girls out and they turned me down flat.

But there is still time. I'm not a bad guy. I'm normal in that way.

I used to get crushes on the nurses in hospital.

Nowadays I'm more outgoing. I'm popular at the shirt factory where I work and I'm a friend of all handicapped and old people.

I spend every spare second raising cash for the League of Friends of Musgrove Park Hospital in Taunton.

It's my way of paying back the medical profession for all they've done for me.'

Andrew's birth should have been the happiest day of her life.

But Mum Vera recalled from the family home in Taunton, Somerset: 'I knew the minute the nurses took him away something was wrong.'

'I saw him and felt sheer bewilderment. It took 10 days to find out what was wrong. It was an enormous hill to climb.'

Andrew suffers from APERTS Syndrome – Accro-Cephalo-Syndactily. And before he helped pioneer the miracle Tessiers operation, victims were unlikely to reach adolescence.

Harley Street paediatrician Dr David Morris said: 'If Andrew had been born a decade earlier, he would probably have died in his teens.'

(Star Sunday Sport, 27 September 1987)

Extract 2.3 Stevenson: 'Treasure island'

Blind Pew

He was plainly blind, for he tapped before him with a stick, and wore a great green shade over his eyes and nose; and he was hunched, as if with age or weakness, and wore a huge old tattered sea-cloak with a hood, that made him appear positively deformed. I never saw in my life a more dreadful looking figure …

I held out my hand, and the horrible, soft-spoken, eyeless creature gripped it in a moment like a vice. I was so much startled that I struggled to withdraw; but the blind man pulled me close to him with a single action of his arm.

(Stevenson, 1883, p.37)

Extract 2.4 Dickens: 'A Christmas carol'

[In the family of Bob Cratchit, clerk to Scrooge, there are several children, one of whom is physically disabled. When we first meet Tiny Tim, he is being carried on his father's shoulder. Mrs Cratchit asks her husband how Tiny Tim behaved when they were out together.]

'As good as gold,' said Bob, 'and better. Somehow, he gets thoughtful, sitting by himself so much, and thinks the strangest things you ever heard. He told me, coming home, that he hoped the people saw him in the church, because he was a cripple, and it might be pleasant for them to remember upon Christmas Day who made lame beggars walk and blind men see.' Bob's voice was tremulous when he told them this, and trembled more when he said that Tiny Tim was growing strong and hearty.

(Dickens, 1843, p.94)

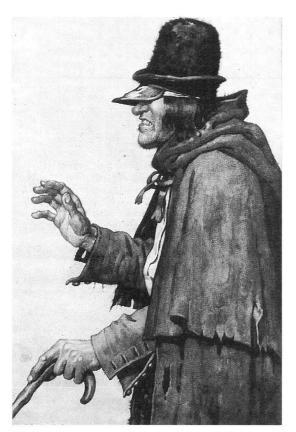

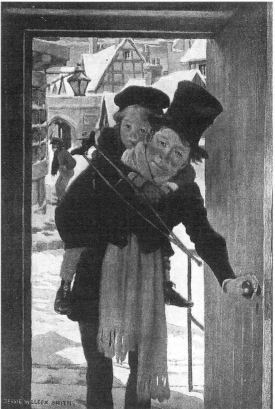

Blind Pew (illustration by Monro S. Orr, 1934)

Bob and Tiny Tim Cratchit on Christmas Day (illustration by Jessie Wilcox Smith, 1925)

Extract 2.5 Evans: 'Pride against prejudice'

[In this extract the disabled woman Pam Evans depicts the multiple stereotypes that confront disabled people in everyday life. Evans presents these stereotypes in a series of bold statements:]

That we feel ugly, inadequate and ashamed of our disability.

That our lives are a burden to us, barely worth living.

That we crave to be 'normal' and 'whole' …

That we are naive and lead sheltered lives.

That we can't ever really accept our condition, and if we appear to be leading a full and contented life, or are simply cheerful, we are 'just putting a good face on it' …

That we desire to emulate and achieve normal behaviour and appearance in all things.

That we go about the daily necessities or pursue an interest because it is a 'challenge' through which we can 'prove' ourselves capable.

That we feel envy and resentment of the able bodied.

That we feel our condition is an unjust punishment.

That any emotion or distress we show can only be due to our disability and not to the same things that hurt and upset them.

That our disability has affected us psychologically, making us bitter and neurotic.

That it's quite amazing if we laugh, are cheerful and pleasant or show pleasure in other people's happiness.

That we are ashamed of our inabilities, our 'abnormalities' and loathe our wheelchairs, crutches or other aids.

That we never 'give up hope' of a cure …

That we are asexual or at best sexually inadequate.

That we cannot ovulate, menstruate, conceive or give birth, have orgasms, erections, ejaculations or impregnate.

That if we are not married or in a long-term relationship it is because no one wants us and not through our personal choice to remain single or live alone.

That if we do not have a child it must be the cause of abject sorrow to us and likewise never through choice.

That any able-bodied person who marries us must have done so for one of the following suspicious motives and never through love: desire to hide his/her own inadequacies in the disabled partner's obvious ones; an altruistic and saintly desire to sacrifice their lives to our care; neurosis of some sort, or plain old fashioned fortune-hunting.

That if we have a partner who is also disabled, we chose each other for no other reason, and not from any other qualities we might possess. When we choose 'our own kind' in this way the able-bodied world feels relieved, until of course we wish to have children; then we're seen as irresponsible …

That if our marriage or relationship fails, it is entirely due to our disability and the difficult person this inevitably makes us, and never from the usual things that make any relationship fail.

That we haven't got a right to an able-bodied partner, and that if they happen to be very obviously attractive, it's even more of a 'waste'.

That any able-bodied partner we have is doing us a favour and that we bring nothing to the relationship.

That we can't actually *do* anything. That we 'sit around' all day 'doing nothing'. Sitting seems to imply resting so it is presumed that we get no 'exercise'.

That those of us whose disability is such that we require a carer to attend to our physical needs are helpless cabbages who don't *do* anything either and have nothing to give and who lead meaningless, empty lives.

That if we are particularly gifted, successful or attractive before the onset of disability our fate is infinitely more 'tragic' than if we were none of these things.

That we should put up with any inconvenience, discomfort or indignity in order to participate in 'normal' activities and events. And this will somehow 'do us good'.

That our only true scale of merit and success is to judge ourselves by the standards of their world.

That our need and right to privacy isn't as important as theirs and that our lives need to be monitored in a way that deprives us of privacy and choice.

That we are sweet, deprived little souls who need to be compensated with treats, presents and praise.

(Evans, quoted in Morris, 1991, pp.19–22)

COMMENT

In Extracts 2.1 and 2.2, the 'human interest' newspaper stories, we have two contrasting yet arguably linked portrayals of what it is to be 'disabled'. In the first there is the 'heroic' individual who is 'part of an extraordinary chess team', extraordinary because 'they are all deaf'. It is not made clear in the story why being a deaf person should make playing chess any more difficult than it is for those who have no hearing impairment. The image is that of the plucky, courageous 'invalid' battling through adversity. By way of contrast the second news story focuses on the tragic, hellish existence of a disabled man who has suffered years of 'cruel taunts' due to his physical appearance. This 'sad' story emphasizes that 'fate has landed him a cruel blow'. This is a narrative or story through which disability is often represented (recall section 2 of Chapter 1, where it was pointed out that social problems are often viewed in terms of people who have problems). However, it also emphasizes again the immense courage and cheerfulness ('27 *years of hell* and he's still *smiling*') of disabled people. In both news stories there is the homogenized portrayal of disabled people as objects of both pity (due to their 'cruel fate') and congratulation (for their 'cheery fortitude'), with differences between people conflated.

In Extracts 2.3 and 2.4 the fictional characters of Blind Pew and Tiny Tim provide us with two contrasting fictional representations of disabled people. On the one hand, Blind Pew is presented as both 'dreadful looking' and viciously evil. Here, Robert Louis Stevenson employs the historically common artistic trick of combining the existence of a physical or sensory impairment with wickedness. We thus have a dramatic association of a person with an impairment being a danger or threat to others (in other words, the deviant as 'bad'). On the other hand, Charles Dickens's portrayal of Tiny Tim is that of the brave and altruistic 'innocent', unsullied by the selfish and materialistic world epitomized by the unreformed Scrooge. Such imagery of disabled people in popular fiction arguably reinforces an 'evil/good' dichotomy vis-à-vis disabled people in the popular imagination. As Morris (1991, p.93) points out, in much popular fiction it is evident that disability is used as 'a metaphor, as a code, for the message that the non-disabled writer wishes to get across in the same way that "beauty" is used'. Morris goes on to contend that when disability is used as a metaphor for evil or strangeness, the stereotype is confirmed.

Finally, in Extract 2.5 Pam Evans adopts the devices of irony and confrontation in her powerful indictment of the prejudiced attitudes towards disabled people that are held by the dominant able-bodied majority in contemporary society. The extract is an ironic chronicle of the multiple levels and contradictory ways in which prejudice operates. By means of its contestation of stereotypes of what it is to be 'disabled', this extract also opens up potentially new opportunities or 'spaces' for understanding the complex and varied experiences of disabled people. To be 'disabled' is not to be one member of a homogeneous group. Instead, Pam Evans offers us the chance to understand disabled people as, for example, women, sexual beings, private citizens, workers, and so on. Taken as a whole this extract challenges the dominant constructions of disability and may be understood as part of the disability movement's questioning and subversion of what was referred to in Chapter 1 as the hegemonic ideology of disablism.

deviant

ideology

■ ■ ■

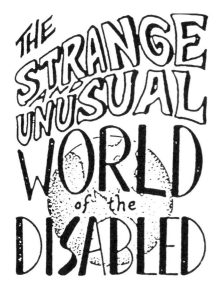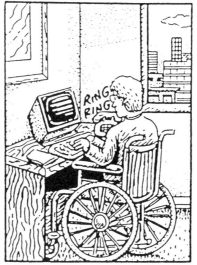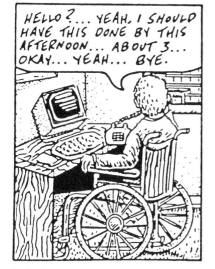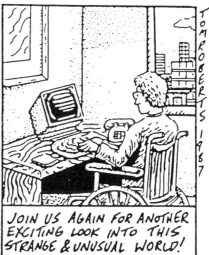

Rethinking disability?

On the basis of Activity 2.1 you will be aware that the popular cultural representations of disability in the UK are historically complex, contradictory and contested, and that disability is not an indivisible category. However, the dominant constructions of disability have arguably established a deviant, and relatively powerless, status for the disabled as other – distinct and apart from the supposedly 'normal' and 'natural' majority. Kurtz's (1981) sociological discussion of dominant images of people with 'mental retardation' offers a valuable contribution to our understanding of the creation of the role of the 'outsider' or the 'other' for people labelled as disabled and thus deviant. Kurtz presents a list of images which illustrate further the power of stereotyping with regard to disabled people – in this case people with learning difficulties – across works of art, religions, popular imagination and 'expert' discourses. According to Kurtz, eight images of the 'mentally retarded' have been historically and cross-culturally dominant:

other

1   as the sub-human organism

2   as the menace with a weak mind in a strong body

3   as the object of pity

4   as the eternal child/holy innocent

5   as the burden of charity

6   as the object of shame

7   as the object of ridicule

8   as the sick person (adapted from Kurtz, 1981).

Kurtz's classification of images of disability itself raises some further questions. You may ask yourself how exhaustive it is.

Could the classification be applied to groups other than people with learning difficulties, for example people with a physical or sensory impairment, people with mental health problems, people with a 'hidden' impairment (such as epilepsy or diabetes), or those with stigmatized conditions such as HIV?

Since the types of impairment associated with disabled people are immense and complex, Kurtz's focus on the dominant stereotypes of people with learning difficulties, who themselves are diverse and differentiated in terms of attributes, skills, etc., is likely to be an inadequate framework for our understanding of the social construction of disabled people in general (even assuming it is possible to speak of such a 'group'). Furthermore, Kurtz's work does not capture the ways in which the stereotyping of marginalized categories of people tends to involve a convergence and combining of negative images. Williams (1992) has noted that negative stereotyping is a common element in the subordination suffered by all oppressed groups. Indeed, stereotypes about women with learning difficulties, for example, are likely to converge with sexist and racist stereotypes, often in highly contradictory ways. Williams (1992, p.151) points out that women with learning difficulties are often subject to contradictory stereotyping, whereby they are seen as both submissive and dangerous, irrational and cunning, innocent and tainted.

Among the powerful and negative popular representations which Kurtz's classification fails to consider are the following:

■   the disabled person as the object of violence

■   the disabled person as sinister and evil

■   the disabled person as atmosphere or curio

■   the disabled person as 'super cripple' or hero

■   the disabled person as 'their own worst enemy' and self-pitying

■   the disabled person as sexually dysfunctional (adapted from Barnes, 1992).

It will be apparent from the discussion so far that there exists a wide-ranging and contradictory repository of images about disabled people in popular culture. For the most part such contradictory images represent disabled people as deviant outsiders in clear juxtaposition to the normal, and thus naturalized, 'able-bodied' **marginalization** majority. Marginalization is the term used by social scientists to describe this complex process of the social exclusion of deviant groups such as disabled people from the dominant culture.

Despite the contribution of sociologists such as Kurtz to the understanding of the dominant popular constructions of disability, it would be misleading to absolve social science from the marginalization, neglect and distortion of disabled people as the deviant 'other'. In Chapter 1 we saw how social science perspectives also become sedimented as 'traces' in common sense. Only since the early 1990s, and largely due to the work of disabled activists and sociologists such as Mike Oliver in the UK, has social science in general and sociology in particular begun seriously to theorize and research disability as a social phenomenon and contest the dominant medical discourse on disability (to which we return in section 6). Oliver argues:

> The issue of disability and the experiences of disabled people have been given scant consideration in academic circles. Both the issue and the experience have been marginalized and only in the disciplines of medicine and psychology has disability been afforded an important place. Unfortunately this has, itself, been counter-productive because it has resulted in the issue of disability being seen as essentially a medical one and the experience of disability as being contingent upon a variety of psychological adjustment processes. Hence there is an urgent need for other disciplines such as sociology, anthropology, history, politics and social administration to take these matters seriously rather than to merely offer descriptive and atheoretical accounts which leave medical and psychological approaches unchallenged.
>
> (Oliver, 1990, pp.x–xi)

Oliver's critique both of the dominant medical and psychological models of disability and of existing limited work in such disciplines as sociology, social administration and history shows that academic knowledge is culpable in contributing to the wider marginalization and distortion of the experiences of disabled people noted above. Oliver's critique also illustrates that social scientific knowledge itself is forever contested and subject to controversy.

Summary

This section has introduced you to some of the key contemporary and historical representations of disability. We have concentrated largely on popular cultural representations of disability as a result of which disabled people become classified as the deviant outsider, abnormal and unnatural when compared to the assumed normal and natural insider, the able-bodied. However, we have also seen that to be a disabled person is not to be part of a unitary or natural 'condition' untouched by social context and changing constructions. In passing we may note that the nature and meaning of 'able-bodied' remains largely untheorized, unmentioned and most importantly unproblematized in common sense, except in radical challenges to the dominant constructions such as we saw in Extract 2.5. We shall examine this further in section 6. Finally, this section has suggested that academic social science has also tended to marginalize the study of disability and thus accept the dominant medical model of disability on which we focus in section 5.

normal/abnormal
natural/unnatural

3   What is disability? Some 'definitions', 'facts' and 'figures'

It will not have escaped you that so far we have not situated the discussion in the 'hard' ground of facts and figures about the nature and extent of disability in the UK. It is not that questions such as 'how much disability is there?' or 'how might one measure disability?' are insignificant to social scientific analysis. Rather, the quest for such quantifiable certainties may prove a futile endeavour in any attempt to understand the socially constructed character of disability. Let us first explore the problem of defining disability.

3.1   Defining disability

Chapter 1 has alerted you to the different, often competing, definitions and constructions of poverty among social scientists. In this section we will explore the difficulties in attempting to provide an uncontested definition of disability. As the chapter progresses, you may be able to arrive at your own preferred working definition of the term disability. However, as you will see from Activity 2.2 below, we shall be treating disability as a contested concept and therefore open to competing definitions of its 'nature'.

ACTIVITY 2.2

Think carefully about what disability means to you, and try to define it. Then compare your definition with those given below.

The definition of a phenomenon is of course crucial for any subsequent attempt to investigate its nature and to measure its extent in society. The definition of disability used by social scientists will profoundly influence how they approach its analysis, as you saw with the example of poverty in Chapter 1. Bear this point in mind when you read the following definitions. As you read them, consider the positive or negative assumptions that are embedded in each. You should also consider the extent to which the definitions carry different policy connotations and whether they see disability as a political issue or as an individualistic and medical problem.

- Definition 1 (*Collins Concise English Dictionary*, 1986): '(1) the condition of being unable to perform a task or function because of a physical or mental impairment; (2) something that disables; handicap; (3) lack of necessary intellect, strength etc.; (4) an incapacity in the eyes of the law to enter into certain transactions'.

- Definition 2 (*Concise Oxford Dictionary of Sociology*, 1994): 'Loss or lack of functions, either physical or mental, such as blindness, paralysis or mental subnormality – which unlike illness, is usually permanent. Disabilities are usually stigmatising. Moreover, disabled persons often need extra finances and personal support (which is often inadequate to sustain their rights) and are a key group in social security and welfare programmes'.

- Definition 3 (from the British Disability Discrimination Act 1995): 'A person has a disability if he or she has a physical or mental impairment which has a *substantial and long-term* adverse effect on his or her ability to carry out normal day-to-day activities'.

- Definition 4 (from Union of the Physically Impaired Against Segregation (UPIAS), in Rieser and Mason, 1990, p.87):

  Impairment – lacking all or part of a limb, organ or mechanism of the body.

  Disability – the disadvantage or restriction of activity caused by a contemporary social organisation which takes no or little account of people who have physical impairments and thus excludes them from the mainstream of social activities – physical disability is therefore a particular form of social oppression.'

- Definition 5 (from Driedger, 1989): '*Disability* is the functional limitation within the individual caused by physical, mental or sensory *impairment*. *Handicap* is the loss or limitation of opportunities to take part in the normal life of the community on an equal level with others due to physical or social barriers.'

- Definition 6 (from Fulcher, a political scientist, 1989, p.21): 'Disability is a category which is central to how welfare states regulate an increasing population of their citizens. In this sense and context, it is a political and social construction used to regulate.'

COMMENT

Definition 1 is overwhelmingly focused on issues of inability and a lack of something in the individual, with a legal link which also focuses on a negative characteristic. Similarly, Definition 2 places most emphasis on the problem of loss or lack, although it does highlight the association of disability with social stigma and the 'dependent' nature of many disabled people on welfare/state provision, thus showing a clear political connotation. Definition 3 is again clear and focused, but is radically different to Definition 2. It offers a medical and individualistic model of disability, thus arguably constructing a notion of normality as natural and taken-for-granted. Definition 4 distinguishes two dimensions (impairment and disability) and, in sharp contrast to Definition 3, the focus is on external (and in a general sense political) institutional oppression (rather than any lack of something in the individual). Even this definition is limited, however, in that it only addresses physical disability. Definition 5 again employs two distinctions, 'disability' and 'handicap'. In this sense it is similar to Definition 4, but in its use of terminology it offers virtually a reversal of the terms used in Definition 4. In contrast to the first five definitions, Definition 6 is extremely abstract and suggests that the category of disability is about the political and institutional regulation of populations. Finally, and perhaps in contrast to your own definition of disability, you may have noticed that all these definitions appear to ignore the idea that disability/able-bodiedness may be seen as a continuum rather than as discrete states.

■ ■ ■

It is clear, then, that there are competing positions as to how disability is best defined. You will have noted how some definitions both assume 'normality' as natural and take for granted the external environment in which people live. There are also differences in the breadth and depth of the definitions. Perhaps most strikingly, the definitions carry very different emphases and assumptions; for example, some stress the 'unable' or impaired individual, while others point to institutions which dis-able people.

Attempting to define disability is therefore a highly problematic business. However, it is not our concern here to judge which is the 'correct' or 'most truthful' definition. Instead, as students of social science, we are more interested in exploring the question of why there are such different constructions of disability and what the implications are of such constructions. It is important to note that language, in this case a series of definitions, is 'a site of struggle and conflict where power relations are acted out and contested' (Burr, 1995, p.41).

3.2 Measuring disability

Let us turn now to consider how the extent of disability has been measured in social surveys. The state-run Office of Population Censuses and Surveys (OPCS) undertook a major research project into the extent of disability in the UK through surveys carried out in both 1968 and 1988. Disabled people were defined as being those who were 'severely or appreciably incapacitated'. The notion of impairment used in both surveys was that of an abnormality in function, with the nature of the external environment taken for granted. The 1968 survey was based on criteria involving self-care (in other words, the extent to which the individual is able to care for him-/herself) and was restricted to the 16+ age group in private households. The survey concluded that there were an estimated 1,128,000 disabled people out of a total population of 53 million.

Other researchers have argued that these first OPCS figures were an underestimate. Townsend's (1967) research focused on the 10+ age group and initially came up with an estimate of three times as many people who were 'severely or appreciably incapacitated' compared to the 1968 OPCS survey. Townsend then reduced his estimate to twice as many disabled people when he removed from his data those respondents who did not specify the disabling condition.

The 1988 OPCS survey employed a different measurement of disability to the 1968 survey; it covered people with all types of disability – physical, sensory and mental. It defined impairment as abnormality in function, disability as not being able to perform an activity considered normal for human beings, and handicap as the inability to perform a normal social role (Oliver, 1990, p.4). The survey also included children and people in institutions. The findings of this research were that there were 5.8 million adults in private households, 400,000 adults in residential institutions, and 360,000 children in private and residential care. This estimate was double that of the previous highest estimate.

Table 2.1 shows some different estimates of the prevalence of disability in the UK since 1968.

Table 2.1   Different estimates of the prevalence of disability

	Number
OPCS, 1968 (GB)	1,128,000
Townsend, 1967 (UK)	3,095,000
Townsend, 1967 (UK)	1,935,000
Outset, 1983 (UK)	2,065,926
Social Services Register, 1982–83 (UK)	1,333,494
OPCS, 1988 (GB)	6,560,000

Source: based on Lonsdale, 1990, p.18

It is questionable whether we could ever know the 'true' extent of disability, given, among other things, the contested nature of its definition, the diversity of types of impairment, difficulties of classification, and also the problem that people have mixed views about defining themselves as 'disabled'. Our discussion confirms the importance of the practice of systematic scepticism which Chapter 1 describes as being an essential feature of social science. This rule applies not least in the refusal to accept self-proclaimed truths from social scientists themselves.

ACTIVITY 2.3

The OPCS research discussed above involved the use of a structured interview schedule, carried out in a face-to-face situation. Selected questions from this interview schedule are reproduced in Table 2.2. In reading these questions, bear in mind the following points:

1   What approach is evident with regard to the problems that disabled people face?

2   What issues may be hidden or neglected by the nature of the questions asked?

Table 2.2   Selected questions from survey of disabled adults, OPCS, 1988

Can you tell me what is wrong with you?

What complaint causes you difficulty in holding, gripping or turning things?

Are your difficulties in understanding people mainly due to a hearing problem?

Do you have a scar, blemish or deformity which limits your daily activities?

Have you attended a special school because of a long-term health problem or disability?

Does your health problem/disability mean that you need to live with relatives or someone else who can help to look after you?

Did you move here because of your health problem/disability?

How difficult is it for you to get about your immediate neighbourhood on your own?

Does your health problem/disability prevent you from going out as often or as far as you would like?

Does your health problem/disability make it difficult for you to travel by bus?

Does your health problem/disability affect your work in any way at present?

Source: Oliver, 1990, p.7

Now look at Table 2.3, which comprises a list of questions drawn up by Mike Oliver as an alternative way of finding out about disability in the UK today. Compare these questions with those contained in the OPCS survey.

Table 2.3   Alternative questions on disability

Can you tell me what is wrong with society?

What defects in the design of everyday equipment like jars, bottles and tins causes you difficulty in holding, gripping or turning them?

Are your difficulties in understanding people mainly due to their inabilities to communicate with you?

Do other people's reactions to any scar, blemish or deformity you may have, limit your daily activities?

Have you attended a special school because of your education authority's policy of sending people with your health problem or disability to such places?

Are community services so poor that you need to rely on relatives or someone else to provide you with the right level of personal assistance?

What inadequacies in your housing caused you to move here?

What are the environmental constraints which make it difficult for you to get about in your immediate neighbourhood?

Are there any transport or financial problems which prevent you from going out as often or as far as you would like?

Do poorly-designed buses make it difficult for someone with your health problem/disability to use them?

Do you have problems at work because of the physical environment or the attitudes of others?

Source: Oliver, 1990, p.8

COMMENT

The two sets of questions clearly reflect different approaches to the nature and extent of disability. As Oliver (1990, pp.7–8) notes, the questions in Table 2.2 focus on the problems that disabled people face due to what are perceived as their own personal inadequacies or functional limitations. Those in Table 2.3, on the other hand, locate the causes of disability as lying within the 'external' physical and social environments.

The attempt to define and measure disability may be seen as an important task for social scientists. However, such efforts may at times be viewed as an attempt to delude ourselves that disability is finite, 'out there' and someone else's problem. Indeed, the classification system embedded in the law and used by the state has been seen by critics like Finkelstein (1985) as a means of reinforcing medical and administrative approaches to disability.

■ ■ ■

Summary

This section has demonstrated the contested nature of social scientific analyses, through the example of one social issue, namely disability. We have noted the contested nature of attempts to define and thus construct disability, and how different definitions carry underlying assumptions about 'appropriate' forms of social intervention. We then focused on research which attempted to measure the extent of disability in the population. This social scientific investigation was seen to be problematic in that its 'objective' findings were necessarily 'contaminated' by their assumptions about the nature of disability and how best to investigate it as a social problem and how to intervene in policy terms. Social scientific research is thus itself part of the wider social construction of disability and is capable of being critically interrogated as a way of knowing about social issues.

4 Religious and moral constructions of disabled people

We noted in section 2 that there is a plethora of common-sense images and stereotypes of disability in contemporary society. In the study of social problems and social divisions it is important to trace in more detail the historical roots of such images – how they become realized and how they are challenged in both the practices of major institutions and in everyday experiences and social encounters.

common sense

4.1 Religious constructions of disability

All the main world religions have passed moral judgement on disability (Miles, 1995). We shall take Judaism and Christianity as our examples, and begin by looking at a passage from the Old Testament as an illustration of religious and moral constructions of disability:

> And the Lord said to Moses, 'Say to Aaron, None of your descendants throughout their generations who has a blemish may approach to offer the bread of his God. For no one who has a blemish shall draw near, a blind man or lame, or one who has a mutilated face or a limb too long, or a man who has an injured foot or an injured hand, or a hunchback or a dwarf, or a man with a defect in his sight or an itching disease or scabs or crushed testicles.'
>
> (Leviticus 21: 16–20)

In this passage, the sense of moral censure of disability is extremely strong, for example in the link between 'blemish' and 'impurity'. The above biblical message about disabled people is that they are tainted/impure persons who pollute the world (and in passing we should note that the same notion of impurity was applied to all women in the Old Testament). A clear link is drawn between deviance and danger. Thomas (1971, p.125) has argued that in most pre-modern societies, disability has been religiously explained as divine punishment for sin/unnatural acts which have produced the 'unnatural being'. The likely response to such happenings was punishment or ostracism. As a result of such religious constructions, the disabled person is considered or 'constituted' as not just 'different' but clearly 'differentiated' and 'deviant'. Here we may note the contemporary resonance with the stigma attached to people with HIV, which has on occasions taken a religious form. Recall the argument in Chapter 1 that representations are crucial in the very constitution of people who are the 'subjects' of such discourses.

Common-sense beliefs about disability as embedded in religious doctrines such as Judaism and Christianity are unlikely to be one-dimensional. Powerful, affective social ideologies often have contradictory appeals in order to function in ordering the world for their subjects. In turn, 'common senses' are most often an untidy 'hotchpotch' or jumbled mixture of elements, with their power residing in their contradictory appeals rather than any logical or rigorous consistency. For example, historically there has not been one simple message about disability in Christianity or in other world religions.

Alongside notions of the disabled as the unnatural, dangerous and deviant 'other', we find in Christianity a moral call to do 'good works' and show pity towards those 'less fortunate'. There is also a strong tradition in Roman Catholicism which encourages a view of disabled people, particularly those with learning difficulties, as somehow 'pure' and 'unsullied' by the temptations of the carnal and material world – 'holy innocents' in the words of Roman Catholic theology. Indeed, this construction of the disabled person as the object of pity and Christian-inspired intervention or 'rescue' lies at the root of many modern charities.

The influence of religiously inspired notions of disability has pervaded what is often regarded as the increasingly secular view of the modern world. Thus the notion of disability as carrying a stigma and being associated with some curse or wickedness is not confined to cultures in the distant past. Common-sense reactions to disability have continued to stigmatize disabled people as 'unnatural' into the twentieth century; this is further confirmation of the importance of 'sediments' and 'traces' in the operation of specific ideologies of normality discussed in Chapter 1.

The discussion so far has concentrated on the theological expression of ideas about what we now term disability. As such we have perhaps run the risk of artificially separating out ideas from the practices of people and institutions. It is important to note, however, that ideas do not exist somehow detached from the lived realities of people's lives nor outside the institutions in which they are embedded. We should therefore look at the complex articulation and re-working of religiously based notions of disability in the major specialist institutions for managing disabled people in recent UK history, namely the charities.

4.2   From construction to intervention: charities and the emergence of the dominant institutional response to disability

The early history of charities for disabled people is essentially linked to the religious and moralistic constructions of disability discussed above. The explicitly religious roots of many charities continue to be manifest in the rationale and procedures of those Western charities that operate throughout the world. Thus, for example, Christian Aid remains one of the largest world-wide charities. However, the discourses of most charities since the nineteenth century are also tied to notions of disabled people as medical problems, who, if not curable, need to be 'helped' or 'subjected' to particular regimes of 'moral management', discipline and segregation. It is therefore difficult to disentangle charitable and medical models of disability, as they have been mutually supportive since the mid to late nineteenth century.

The experiences of disabled people both in charity institutions and outside in the community have been largely hidden from public view. However, in the 1990s there have been attempts to research this forgotten history by means of the oral history of disabled people speaking for themselves.

ACTIVITY 2.4

Memories and recollections are a particularly important source of historical data about the nature of the lived experiences of oppressed groups whose lives have been 'hidden from history'. Read the account by David Swift of his childhood in Extract 2.6, introduced by Humphries and Gordon (1992), and try to unpack the common-sense constructions described in the passage, paying particular attention to the following features:

- religious imagery
- negative popular stereotypes
- the isolation of disabled people in the supposedly 'normal' community.

Extract 2.6 Swift: 'A Nottingham childhood'

David Swift was born in 1936, the son of a miner. He was brought up with his two elder brothers and sister on a council estate on the outskirts of Nottingham. In many ways he was very similar to the other boys on the estate. He collected cigarette cards, he read the *Hotspur* comic, he kept rabbits, he was a passionate Notts County supporter and he loved swinging through the trees pretending he was Tarzan. But in one important respect David was very different from most of the other children. From birth he had an hereditary muscular disease. As a result he walked with a pronounced limp and he found it increasingly difficult to co-ordinate his finger and thumb movements …

> My grandma used to say that I'd been cursed and that I was being punished by God for what I'd done in a past life. That was why I was disabled she said, and when I'd served out this punishment everything would be all right. I used to wonder what it was I'd done so bad to make me like this. I felt as if, well, if I'm cursed I ought to be aware of why, didn't I? But I had no idea what it could be. Nobody seemed to care … I felt as though I were different, like a freak in a side show. I remember when we all used to go to Nottingham Goose Fair and they used to have side shows and all the freaks would lay there. And I always remember thinking to myself, I wonder if I should sit up there with my feet showing? You know and people pay sixpence a time, coming in and looking at my feet. There was nobody else around like me was there? There was nowhere else I could go. I used to have this great fear that they would get rid of me or put me down because I was disabled. Fathers used to take cats and drown them in the river and I used to think that's the way they would do it to me, that's the way they killed you. We had a dog called Pete and he broke his leg. So they decided to have him destroyed and I used to think, well, why destroy dogs that can walk on three legs? I thought, perhaps they put human beings down as well, perhaps they'll destroy me, because I can't walk? I used to spend a lot of time on my own in the graveyard. I used to ponder over all the things that you saw on the gravestones you know. I used to think, I wonder if God needs me more than they, I wonder if God's wanting me? I didn't want God to want me, I was too young. I wanted to stay on this earth. I had this constant fear that they were going to get me. I didn't want to die.
>
> (Humphries and Gordon, 1992, pp.11–12)

Now read Extract 2.7 by Mary Baker, who in 1935 was sent to the Halliwick House for Crippled Girls, a Church of England institution for physically and mentally disabled girls. Mary Baker's impairment was a dislocated hip, which meant she walked with a limp. When her mother died, the authorities decided that her father would not be able to care for Mary and her three brothers.

What are the main features of the segregative institutional life that Mary encountered at Halliwick House? Try to compare her experiences with the visual 'message' about institutional life conveyed in the photograph below.

Extract 2.7 Baker: 'An institutionalized childhood'

When I first arrived at Halliwick the nurse took me into this bathroom and she stripped me off completely. She cut my hair short, right above the ears. And then I was deloused with powder of some description. Then they put me in a bath and scrubbed me down with carbolic soap. It was very degrading to me. And I felt as though the end of the world had come and so I cried, I sat in the bath and cried my eyes out. At any rate they told me it was no good in crying and dried me down. They used such rough towels it felt like they were sandpapering me. Then I was dressed in the Halliwick uniform, navy blue socks, stockings and a gym slip and a serge jumper and I was taken up into the dormitory, a big huge room it seemed, with about ten beds in it. I went in there and lay down on my new bed. I felt awful and I thought that nobody cared for me. Anyway, I don't think that I slept that night, I felt so lonely …

I had entered a different life. My father was far back home and I thought that everyone had forsaken me. I think I cried most of the night. So this was my start. The next morning you were given a number and you had to remember it. My number was twenty-nine and when I got up and went to wash, my towel and flannel had my number on them. Twenty-nine was engraved on all my hairbrushes and things with a big hot poker like thing. Everything I owned had a marking of twenty-nine on, so I can never forget that number. Our lockers in the playroom had the same number and our clothes were marked with our numbers, so we knew what we had. We were hardly ever called by our first names, only by the other girls. And if matron wanted you she called you by twenty-nine or whatever number you had. We never had names, we were just numbers there. It was all very disciplined. I couldn't make it out at first, why we should all have numbers and not names. I felt a bit low about it. I couldn't really put my feelings into an expression, only that I felt very lonely about it.

(Humphries and Gordon, 1992, pp.68–9)

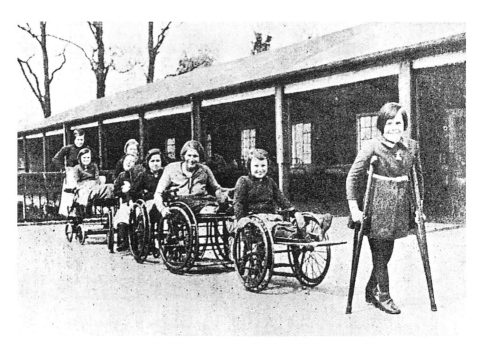

This photograph was used on the front cover of the January 1938 edition of Brothers and Sisters, *a monthly magazine produced by the Children's Union; the smiling faces of the children mask the harshness of many institutions for disabled children*

COMMENT

In the extract by David Swift it is evident that disability in the 1940s and 1950s continued to be surrounded by ignorance, fear and superstition, feeding off religious as well as superstitious notions of blame and the 'sub-human nature' of disabled people that continued well into the twentieth century in the UK. In the account there is evidence of the notion that the birth of a disabled child was viewed commonsensically as a form of 'divine retribution'. Indeed, there is a clear indication that David Swift's impairment was viewed as a curse on the family and in turn led to the construction of the deeply troubled personality of the isolated young man.

In the photograph opposite we are offered a representation of disabled children as happy, appreciative, clean, full of gratitude and 'captured' in an orderly parade. Such a representation contrasts with the grim realities of the institution of the special school described in Mary Baker's recollections, in which strict regimentation, impersonal control and what Goffman (1961) has characterized sociologically as 'institutional dehumanization' dominate. In such institutions all aspects of life are conducted in the same place, all activities are done in the company of a large number of people, all people are required to do the same thing together, and all parts of the day's activities are routinely and tightly scheduled and controlled by officials. The consequence for the inmate is institutionalization and a resultant loss of sense of self. Indeed, most special schools run by charities appear to have been organized on the principles of mechanical obedience, uniformity and the habits of hard work (see the photographs below). Such strict disciplinary regimes were of course a feature of all Victorian institutions of treatment and correction.

■ ■ ■

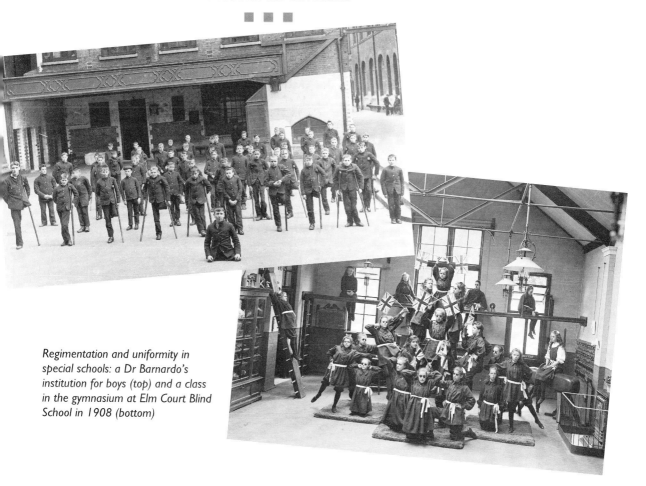

Regimentation and uniformity in special schools: a Dr Barnardo's institution for boys (top) and a class in the gymnasium at Elm Court Blind School in 1908 (bottom)

Since the 1970s there has been a decline in charitable regimes based on institutional segregation. However, charities retain a crucial role in both the representation of what is disability and in the organization of the mixed economy of 'care' for disabled people. In terms of their work and size of operation, charities in the UK today are big business. For example, managerial texts are now available on such topics as *Meeting Need: Successful Charity Marketing* (Bruce, 1994) and *Managing Charitable Investments* (Harrison, 1994). In 1990 there were 170,000 registered charities in the UK. In the same year the top 200 charities had a combined voluntary income of £1 billion, and of these top 200, 50 per cent were medicine and health charities (Hevey, 1992, p.18).

One of the main ways in which charities make money is through advertising. Thus the images of disability that are held by the public are predominantly derived from charity advertisements. Nevertheless, as was suggested in section 2, disability generally remains a taboo topic.

Study the advertisements from the late 1980s and early 1990s shown opposite. Focus on both the written text and the visual representation of disabled people in each advertisement. In your view, what message is conveyed in terms of the following:

■ the situation of disabled people in society

■ the nature of the disability

■ the future life chances of the disabled people in question

■ the role of the charity in question.

Note also the names of the charities. What clues do they give regarding the rationale and routine procedures of many charities in the late twentieth century?

COMMENT

There is probably no one definitive reading of such advertisements, although you will probably agree that the imagery and the written messages are very powerful. When we look 'into' each advertisement it is often possible to see the articulation of both identities and interventions in accordance with the medical classification of conditions. The charities, as institutions, are portrayed as altruistic enterprises established to take care of disabled people. Much of the overall thrust of the messages appears to be an attempt to engender pity and guilt. As Hevey (1992) notes, there is a medical and dependency view of disability embedded in such representations as Mencap's 'A Mental Handicap Is There For Life. So is Mencap' (a poster) and the Multiple Sclerosis Society's 'It's much easier for you to make a stand against Multiple Sclerosis' (an advertisement). Hevey goes on to contend that such advertisements present a view of disabled people in which impairment and the disability are contained *within* the body, and that through such advertisements disabled persons exist as 'a voiceless, powerless hyper-presence within charity funding'. As a consequence, Hevey contends that charity advertising may be viewed as 'the visual flagship for the myth of the tragedy of impairment' (Hevey, 1992, pp.51–2). Even those disabled people seemingly in mainstream society, as in the advertisement for the British Diabetic Association, are presented as being the sufferers of a hidden but tragic fate, casting a 'shadow' over even young lives.

■ ■ ■

*Charity advertisements from
the late 1980s/early 1990s
(Source: The Multiple
Sclerosis Society, Mencap
and the British Diabetic
Association)*

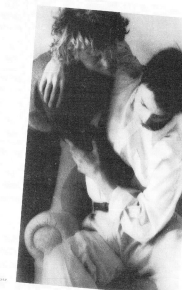

It's much
easier for you
to make a
stand against
Multiple Sclerosis.

MS
Tears lives apart

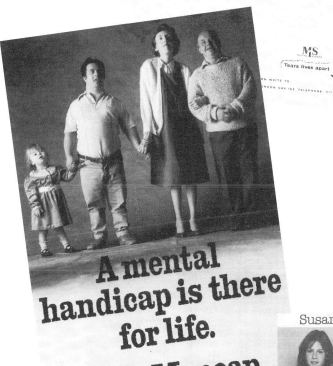

A mental
handicap is there
for life.
So is Mencap.

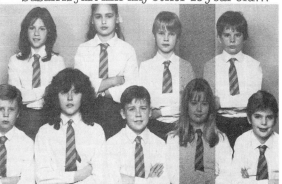

Susan is just like any other 10 year old...

but she lives under
the shadow of diabetes.

*THE SHADOW
OF DIABETES*

BRITISH DIABETIC ASSOCIATION
10 Queen Anne Street London W1M 0BD Telephone: 01-323 1531

It could be argued that charity advertising relies heavily on what may be termed the 'pity button': drawing on traditional perceptions of being in need of help and being the object of both guilt and pity, together with the portrayal of disabled people as being personally tragic and/or dependent and eternal children. Coexisting with such appeals is the theme of benevolent humanitarianism which (paternalistically) expects the clients to be grateful recipients. As Fulcher (1989, p.29) notes, the sources of such assumptions are to be found in the 'hierarchical politics' of the Victorian era, in which the 'deserving poor' were expected to be suitably grateful for any charity dispensed by their social superiors.

Why might a strategy of charity advertising based on pity and fear be adopted?

It may be contended that such a strategy is employed because 'it works' in terms of generating funds. The assumptions of many charities appear to be that there may be a pragmatic need to use the 'pity button'. In understanding this position, it should be noted that under UK law a charity must be apolitical, and people who are classified as 'recipients' of its services may not sit on the council of management. In formal terms, a charity must not be a political pressure group. As a 1989 British government White Paper on charities stated: 'The powers and purposes of a charity should not include the power to bring pressure to bear on the government to adopt, to alter or to maintain a particular line of action.' Furthermore, the pragmatism of most charities may be understood from the evidence that the media play an active and selecting role in pressing the claims of certain charities over others, particularly the 'cuddly charities' (medical, animal and child-related) (research cited in *The Guardian*, 'Society' section, 17 April 1996). In a market-driven society, 'selling the product' (including funding for charities for disabled people) may be 'a necessary evil'.

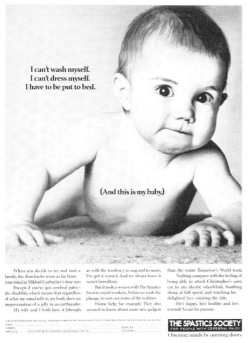

Changing the image: charity advertisements from the mid and late 1990s

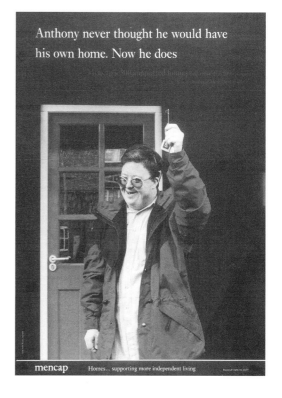

These assumptions run counter to Hevey's claim that there is a need for politicization over the issue of rights versus charity. According to Hevey, there is a struggle between disabled people and what he terms the 'impairment charities'. Underlying this struggle is the argument that charities are 'by far the largest producers and distributors of oppressive/negative disability imagery', with their 'impairment-fixation problem-in-the-body imagery' (Hevey, 1992, p.12). It is important to note that by the mid 1990s some charities became aware of the potential stereotyping and negative imagery associated with the representations of disability carried in advertisements. The advertisements opposite from The Spastics Society (which changed its name to Scope in the mid 1990s) and Mencap are indicative of this growing sensitivity to the criticisms of the messages carried in dominant representations of disability.

It may be argued (Bury, 1996) that the active disability rights and self-advocacy lobby which Hevey supports, just like the charities lobby, may itself be a selective 'voice' of the disabled population, tending not to involve the great majority of disabled people, such as the non-active and chronic disabled elderly. We return to this debate in section 6.

Summary

The above discussion has attempted both to convey and question the dominant common-sense claims about disability. In these dominant constructions of the past and present, disability has been understood and explained as being the reflection of 'naturally occurring distinct types of human beings (Burr, 1995, p.3). In much of the imagery described in this section, disability undergoes what we may term a process of both 'naturalization' and 'simplification'. In other words, there is a powerful appeal to the idea that there is a natural way for disabled people to behave and be responded to, while at the same time the complex nature of what it is to be disabled in some way is dramatically simplified in terms of the dichotomy between 'able-bodied' and 'disabled'. Thus, despite contestations and struggles, disability in the common senses explored above has become what Bannister (1981) has described as a 'nothing but' construction. Seen in this light, disability in common-sense terms ('what everybody knows') is often represented as a fixed, often divinely ordained state of being which in turn has an all-encompassing or global influence on the life of the disabled person (Davidson, 1994). As a consequence of such dominant constructions, disabled people have been subjected to specific policies and practices, historically organized chiefly around institutional segregation and charity.

Much of the history of disability in the UK thus revolves around the dominant belief in the permanent nature of 'handicaps' and the institutional reliance on voluntary efforts to provide 'relief'. Such interventions assumed a state of 'natural' dependency. However, as the nineteenth century unfolded, such views and practices were increasingly fused with and 'colonized' by medical classifications by means of which mental and physical impairments, 'insanity', and unacceptable behaviour such as crime became 'one class of entity namely disease' (Potts, 1982, p.6). The following section examines the nature of and the process by which this medical discourse became the dominant 'expert' construction of disability in the nineteenth and twentieth centuries. We thus explore how this medical discourse 'colonizes' common-sense attitudes towards disability. At the same time we need to remember that this medical construction (disability as pathology) is but one example of a wider process which sociologists have termed the 'medicalization' of social problems (Pearson, 1974).

5   The discourse of disability as pathology: the medical model

discourse

medical model

In Chapter 1 you were introduced to the concept of discourse, which is a crucial concept in the social constructionist approach to the study of social problems. In this section we will examine the rise to dominance of a medical model of disability in the last two centuries as a concrete example of an 'expert' discourse which comes to 'own' a 'problem' – in this case a range of physical, sensory and learning impairments. We will thus explore how discourses relate to constructions through the systematic appropriation of a problem. Our discussion will also study the concrete ways in which knowledge (the way of knowing about something) and power (the way of acting on something) are intertwined, for example the diagnosis of certain mental or cognitive characteristics as pathological. We will also focus on the ways in which 'expert' knowledges are

institutional practices

necessarily embedded and realized through specific institutional practices and regimes (such as the hospital, the special school and the asylum). This section focuses on the examples of medical constructions and interventions with regard to mental health and learning difficulties, although it would have been equally appropriate to have used other examples such as physical and sensory impairments.

The influence of medicine on the diagnosis and treatment of disability is impossible to ignore. Medical interventions occur right across the spectrum, from the determination of whether a foetus is impaired through to the death of elderly people from disabling conditions. As Oliver (1990, p.48) notes, much of the involvement of medicine with disabled people is entirely appropriate, such as in the diagnosis of impairment, the treatment of illness occurring independent of disability, and the provision of physical rehabilitation. However, it may be asked why medical doctors are involved in such areas as the assessment of driving ability and the measurement of work capabilities. How did medicine and, subsequently, the allied therapeutic practices (such as physiotherapy, occupational therapy and psychological counselling), institutionalized around 'pathological conditions', become the dominant 'expert' construction of disability today? There are different histories which help us answer this question.

5.1   The rise of the medical model

In north-west Europe in the seventeenth and eighteenth centuries the 'madman' or 'lunatic' was generally regarded as no better than a beast, due to the person's loss of humanity – that is, reason. 'Madness' was thus a form of animality to be 'mastered' by discipline and brutality (Foucault, 1971). Yet by the end of the nineteenth century the terms 'madman' and 'lunatic' were replaced (at least in expert discourses) by 'insanity' and eventually by 'mental illness'. According to Scull (1979, p.16), the big questions that need to be answered are how insanity came to be exclusively defined as an illness, a condition within the sole jurisdiction of the medical profession, and why 'mad doctors' opted for the asylum as the 'home' within which to receive treatment. In answer to these questions, it would appear that the process of medicalization of this particular category of disabled persons was by no means inevitable but instead resulted from power struggles between contesting 'experts' in and knowledges about the management of the 'mad'. Indeed, in the early decades of the nineteenth century, the first asylums were organized on the basis of a philosophy of 'moral management'.

Moral management represented a non-scientific, pragmatic approach based on the management of mental disorder through the establishment of an orderly, moralizing regime. It represented a guardianship model of 'madness', with inmates characterized by child-like dependency and, in turn, the guardians acting *in loco parentis*. Samuel Tuke, who ran the famous Quaker Retreat in York in the early nineteenth century, was the main proponent of 'moral management', and he firmly rejected the appeal of the apparent 'science' of medicine: 'I have happily little occasion for theory since my province is to relate, not only what ought to be done, but also what, in most instances, is actually performed' (Tuke, 1813).

Given its pragmatic and non-scientific character, the philosophy of moral management was, according to Scull (1979), unable to resist those espousing a less modest ideal, such as the new medical men in the early nineteenth century. This philosophy is epitomized in the following statement from the *Journal of Mental Science* (1858, cited in Scull, 1979): 'Insanity is purely a disease of the brain. The physician is now the responsible guardian of the lunatic and must ever remain so.'

The success of medical doctors during this period is a clear example of the rise to power of a new profession. According to the sociologist Elliot Freidson (1970, p.45), 'Any profession bases its claim for its position on the possession of a "skill" so esoteric or complex that non-members of the profession cannot perform the work safely or satisfactorily and cannot evaluate the work properly.' In such statements as that which launched the *Journal of Mental Science,* the power of exclusive professional knowledge was stated and, in the lunatic asylum, was to be given the crucial institutional location required for a 'successful' discourse.

As we noted in section 4.2, the massive impetus for segregative treatment/ control in the asylum during the late nineteenth and twentieth centuries came from the coalition of charitable and medical interventions. During the course of the late nineteenth century, asylums grew and grew until they had become, in Scull's (1979, p.220) words, 'vast receptacles for the confinement of those without hope'. There was indeed 'profit in madness' during the nineteenth century which perhaps parallels contemporary developments in the profitable industry founded upon the care of the elderly. Whether state-sponsored or charity-sponsored, asylums and institutions for disabled people in general have arguably been used primarily as instruments for segregative control.

However, there were contested interpretations of the 'success' of such institutional and medical experiments, even early on in the history of segregative hospitalization of the 'insane'. One critic, John Arlidge, writing in 1859, likened the growing asylums to 'a machine ... a gigantic evil, and figuratively speaking, a manufactory of chronic insanity'. Whatever the criticisms past and present, the institutional base and material consequences of psychiatry as a part of the hegemonic medical discourse on disability lie historically in the asylum and later in the mental hospital.

So far we have suggested that the rise to dominance of a medical discourse on 'madness' in the nineteenth century was neither 'natural' nor inevitable. From its beginnings, medicine had to struggle to 'colonize' the terrain of the treatment of the 'mad'. It is feasible, for example, that a non-medical discourse, such as that of moral management, might have 'won' the power struggle with profoundly different consequences for the treatment of the mentally ill. If we accept this possibility, then the historically constructed and thus contingent/conditional nature of dominant discourses, including 'scientific' ones like medicine, becomes apparent.

5.2   The full flowering of the medical discourse on disability: the example of the Mental Deficiency Act 1913

The medicalization of disability was not of course restricted to those defined as 'lunatics'. By the beginning of the twentieth century, the 'scientific' study of the mind was to make a further 'colonial' conquest – namely those people designated as 'mental defectives'. To take one important example, in the Mental Deficiency Act 1913, four categories of 'mental defective' were legally distinguished for the first time in English law. This was seemingly a sign of the growing scientific sophistication in this area as well being indicative of the close, even collusive, relationship between the law and the new 'science'. The four categories of 'defective' were defined legally as follows:

(a) Idiots; that is to say, persons so deeply defective in mind from birth or from an early age as to be unable to guard themselves against common physical dangers;

(b) Imbeciles; that is to say, persons in whose case there exists from birth or from an early age mental defectiveness not amounting to idiocy, yet so pronounced that they are incapable of managing themselves or their affairs, or, in the case of children, of being taught to do so;

(c) Feeble-minded persons; that is to say, persons in whose case there exists from birth or from an early age mental defectiveness not amounting to imbecility, yet so pronounced that they require care, supervision, and control for their own protection or for the protection of others, or, in the case of children, that they by reason of such defectiveness appear to be permanently incapable of receiving proper benefit from the instruction in ordinary schools;

(d) Moral imbeciles; that is to say, persons who from an early age display some permanent mental defect coupled with strong vicious or criminal propensities on which punishment has had little or no deterrent effect.

(Mental Deficiency Act 1913)

The very use of the term 'deficiency' sends a particular message regarding the innate inferiority and lesser human worth of people thus designated, even accepting the particular historical context in which the classification is located. In the four classifications, 'mental defectives' were categorized in terms of degrees of dependency and danger, both to themselves and others. In terms of the interventionist consequences of such a classification scheme, institutional and segregative care, supervision and control would 'naturally' ensue, authorized by the power of the law. As 'natural' and passive inhabitants of this expertly defined state of being, 'mental defectives' would be subjected to a life of institutionalized dependency with few, if any, rights.

Here we have a striking example of the closely interwoven relationship between medico-scientific knowledge and the legal discourse on 'disability' in the construction of particular categories of people who are systematically differentiated and excluded from the 'healthy' and 'normal' majority.

5.3   Eugenics and the 'threat' of disabled people

The development of a new science for the classification of the human species along a continuum from superior to inferior types is most clearly articulated by the rise of eugenics in Europe and the USA in the early twentieth century. Eugenics lays claim to be the science and study of the methods of improving the quality of the human 'race', especially by means of selective breeding to produce a 'strong race' and thereby avoid the 'contamination' of the 'racial stock' brought by immigrants. According to this body of work, certain 'populations' (for instance 'the poor', other 'alien races', 'the feeble-minded', etc.) were seen as having genetic defects which could not be changed. In turn, such 'defective' and 'dangerous' people were likely to threaten moral values and social order, and in particular they were likely to reproduce more defective people. The notion of mentally, sensorally and physically disabled people as not just an inferior form of humanity but also a dangerous lesser species was clearly in evidence in such legislation as the Mental Deficiency Act of 1913 in Britain and in similar contemporaneous legislation in the USA and Europe.

Eugenics was, and is, arguably less focused on the individual as a subject to be 're-formed' when compared with other medical and 'scientific' interventions. Eugenics was concerned rather with the reorganization and reconstitution of whole populations. This approach reached its lowest point in Nazi Germany, where 400,000 people were subject to compulsory sterilization up to 1939 and, after 1939, as a result of the euthanasia programme, about 200,000 disabled people were killed. This programme also developed the technology for the mass killings of the Jewish and other holocausts (see Proctor, 1988; Morris, 1991).

It should be noted that the appeal of eugenics, particularly the notion that the 'mentally deficient' were an inferior form of human life, was not exclusive to Nazi Germany. In early twentieth-century Britain, John Langdon-Down, the medical superintendent of an asylum, was influential in grouping those people with learning difficulties with supposedly 'primitive' ethnic groups such as 'Mongolian', 'Ethiopian', 'Aztec' and 'Negroid'. According to Langdon-Down, people with learning difficulties inherited the non-European features of those races which could be assumed to be further back on the evolutionary scale and thus more 'animal-like' in nature. Here, then, is a clear example of the 'racialized' construction of disability (see Chapter 3). However, as Hattersley (1987) notes, Langdon-Down intended his work to show the clearly inherited nature of 'sub-normality' in order to help relieve parents and others of any blame or guilt!

Ideas associated with eugenics have continued to resurface in contemporary debates on genetic testing and what was termed the 'new genetics' in the late twentieth century – a development again illustrative of the importance of both change and continuity in the 'story' of disability. The 'new genetics' appears to situate genes as the first cause of various human experiences and behaviour, and tends to assume that human social action is caused by genetic endowment. In criticism, Shakespeare (1995) has noted that the 'old eugenics' and 'new

change and
continuity

genetics' have used supposedly natural characteristics to justify the subordination of oppressed groups such as women, gays and lesbians, black people and disabled people. The term commonly used by social scientists to describe this process is that of 'biological determinism'.

Our discussion of eugenics should have alerted you to the important links between the medical and 'scientific' classification of 'defective' categories of human minds and bodies and the wider processes of social control of 'problem' populations. Put starkly, social constructions at times kill people. You should now be aware how the medical discourse played a significant role in wider ideological debates (beyond disability) about the fears of class unrest, 'racial contamination' and the control of unproductive and 'dangerous' deviants. Furthermore, in the light of our brief discussion of the resurgence of the 'new genetics' in the late twentieth century, you should also be aware that the issues raised by eugenic theories are not of mere antique curiosity value. They have resurfaced in contemporary debates on supposedly 'faulty' bodies, whether they be disabled people or gay men (given the much vaunted discovery of the 'gay gene' – see Chapter 4), or genetic counselling and the pressure on parents in the 1990s to have only 'normal' babies.

5.4   The psychological approach to deviance and disability

Alongside the biological/genetic perspective, the twentieth century has witnessed the growing influence of psychological knowledge with regard to the constructions of both deviance generally and disability in particular. For example, the Wood Committee (1929), an influential expert body, was instrumental in persuading the British state to adopt for the first time the cause of psychology as a crucial instrument in the discovery and treatment of 'mental defectives'. According to this committee, 'on the basis of the best scientific opinion … the real criterion of mental deficiency is a social one, and that a mentally defective individual, whether child or adult, is one who by reason of incomplete mental development is incapable of independent social adaptation' (Wood Committee, 1929, p.152). Despite the use of the term 'social', the definition offered here stresses the importance of psychological factors grouped around the notion of 'intelligence'. The committee, from its position of being at the 'cutting edge' of scientific investigation at the time, went on to criticize existing legislative classifications such as those established in the Mental Deficiency Acts of 1913 and 1927.

As a result of such interventions, the 'new science' of psychology was able to enter the already crowded terrain of expertise on people with impairments. Subsequent decades would see a growth industry in the testing of young people as well as other adult deviants, such as criminals, by a growing army of psychological experts and 'scientists' of the mind.

ACTIVITY 2.7

Read Extract 2.8 from the Mental Health Act 1959. Focus in particular on how 'mental disorder' and 'subnormality' are constructed in medical/psychiatric/ psychological terms, and compare the definitions with those of 'mental deficiency' and 'idiocy' in the quote from the Mental Deficiency Act of 1913 in section 5.2.

Extract 2.8 Mental Health Act 1959: 'Definition and classification of mental disorder'

(1)   In this Act 'mental disorder' means mental illness, arrested or incomplete development of mind, psychopathic disorder, and any other disorder or disability of mind; and 'mentally disordered' shall be construed accordingly.

(2)   In this Act 'severe subnormality' means a state of arrested or incomplete development of mind which includes subnormality of intelligence and is of such a nature or degree that the patient is incapable of living an independent life or of guarding himself against serious exploitation, or will be so incapable when of an age to do so.

(3)   In this Act 'subnormality' means a state of arrested or incomplete development of mind (not amounting to severe subnormality) which includes subnormality of intelligence and is of a nature or degree which requires or is susceptible to medical treatment or other special care or training of the patient.

(4)   In this Act 'psychopathic disorder' means a persistent disorder or disability of mind (whether or not including subnormality of intelligence) which results in abnormally aggressive or seriously irresponsible conduct on the part of the patient, and requires or is susceptible to medical treatment.

(5)   Nothing in this section shall be construed as implying that a person may be dealt with under this Act as suffering from mental disorder, or from any form of mental disorder described in this section, by reason only of promiscuity or other immoral conduct.

(Mental Health Act 1959, Appendix 1, section 4)

COMMENT

This extract from the 1959 Act clearly illustrates the full blossoming of the medical model of mental illness: medical, quasi-technical classifications are presented unproblematically. According to this model, the disability clearly resides in the individual's mind, whether in the shape of a disorder or subnormality. It is thus an individual pathology to be diagnosed and treated by medicine. Here we see an individualistic construction of disability leading logically to medical interventions in terms of individual problems. In order to bolster the objective nature of the disabling 'condition' of mental illness, point (5) of the definition in the 1959 Act alerts us to the need to separate medical issues from moral ones. In contrast, the 1913 Mental Deficiency Act, particularly with regard to 'moral imbeciles', coupled 'mental defect' to 'strong vicious or criminal propensities' and indeed went on to give local authorities powers to place people having sex outside of marriage into institutions. Over the course of five decades, therefore, we see significant changes in emphasis, but also continuities in the mode of analysis adopted in this medical discourse.

■ ■ ■

Following the rise to dominance of this medical discourse on mental illness in the UK in the late 1950s, segregative hospitalization, allied to psychotropic drug 'therapy' and intrusive measures such as electro-convulsive therapy, came to dominate the welfare state's routine treatment of people with mental illness. Such treatment regimes themselves subsequently became subject to criticism both from within and outside the medical establishment in Britain and elsewhere (Sedgwick, 1982). In this context the publication in Britain of the Department of Health and Social Security report *Better Services for the Mentally Ill* (1975) was hailed in mainstream academic and policy circles as a watershed in the treatment of 'the mentally ill' in particular and 'the disabled' in general. Such praise (for example Topliss, 1982) was largely due to the report's concern to seek a 'humane' understanding of the difficulties of people with mental health problems, as the following extract from the report illustrates:

> Mental illness and conversely mental health is notoriously difficult to define. There is now a deep interest in the psychological aspects of human behaviour, collectively as well as individually, an interest which is constantly extending to new facets of everyday life in society …
>
> How do we then define mental illness? On the one hand 'mental illness' as a term probably still has a certain stigma attached to it and most of us probably draw our own fine dividing line between the more comprehensible and respectable forms of mental ill health and the more frightening or distressing forms which we privately label as mental illness. But on this kind of definition the mentally ill would constitute only a small proportion – in practice mainly those with psychotic illness – of the total numbers of those who are currently seeking and receiving help from general practitioners and psychiatrists for psychological problems of various kinds, from severe depression, and phobias, through a whole range of sexual, marital and other human relationship problems. Equally we have to acknowledge that there are many problems of human behaviour – often causing great distress – for which psychiatry can offer little or no remedy and for which other forms of help and support may be more relevant.
>
> (Department of Health and Social Security, 1975, pp.1–2)

Compared to the apparent certainties of classifications and definitions in the nineteenth and early to mid twentieth century (see Activity 2.7 above), the tenor of this report is much more guarded about the rigidity of both the definition and extent of mental illness. At the same time, the key role of psychiatry and medicine in the diagnosis and treatment of such an 'illness' is clearly reaffirmed. It would also seem to represent a further acknowledgement of the growing ascendancy of a (social) psychological model of mental illness within the overarching medical discourse on disability. Accordingly, the new knowledge evident in the passage establishes the possibility of an ever-expanding population of subjects suffering in varying ways and to varying degrees from this 'illness'.

Our discussion of some of the major continuities and transformations in the dominant medical discourse on 'mental deficiency' and 'mental illness' in the twentieth century may well have alerted you to a seeming paradox. This paradox relates to the coexistence of clear continuities and apparent discontinuities in how both 'mental illness' and 'subnormality' were to be understood and treated by the scientific medical expert. However, this paradox may be more imagined than real. Remember that Chapter 1 argued that discourses are neither static nor totally stable. Discourses themselves, as well as the subjects of their practices, have a history that is often complex and messy. Our discussion of the medical constructions of and interventions directed towards people with learning difficulties and people with mental health problems will have provided you with some concrete illustrations of this broader 'truth'.

5.5   From institutional segregation to 'community treatment'

The latest phase in the policy response to the 'problem' of disabled people in the UK in the twentieth century was the much heralded shift from institutional care to community care after the 1970s, epitomized by the National Health and Community Care Act of 1990 and 'community care' provisions implemented after 1993. Any detailed examination of this trend in policy and practice is beyond the remit of this chapter. It suffices at this point to note that different, contested constructions of disability (both medical and non-medical) underpinned 1990s debates on community care. Furthermore, there are important links between the shifting definitions or knowledges of, in this case, disability and the institutionalized practices of welfare.

In the UK in the 1970s and 1980s, people once regarded variously as 'idiots', 'mongols', 'retarded', 'mentally deficient', 'subnormal', 'mentally impaired', 'mentally handicapped', etc. were increasingly seen as having 'special needs' or 'learning difficulties' in policy and professional circles. The concept of learning difficulty arose from a new understanding that 'subnormal' people were educable. This view was intellectually and institutionally embedded in the Warnock Report (1978) and the subsequent Education Act (1980). The philosophy of 'special needs' was keen to promote the integration of people into ordinary life, to make them more independent and to equip them with various social and practical skills. Critics have pointed out that this approach focused on individual difference and lack of ability, which often meant that provision of services remained separate from the 'mainstream'. Special needs assessment remained based on medical, psychological and educational advice. There was also an assumption that there was a fixed percentage of children who were likely to be in need. It might be argued that the terms 'special needs' and 'learning difficulties' have become pejorative labels attached to disabled people (Quicke, 1985, p.7).

What is perhaps most interesting for our purposes is the changing language of the debate on people with learning difficulties over the decades of the late twentieth century. We are again confronted by the issue of how new and emergent 'expert' discourses come to 'own' a problem through the creation and subsequent institutionalization of powerful knowledges about that problem. Just how long the term 'people with learning difficulties' will retain its currency is difficult to forecast in the late twentieth century, but the fate of previous constructions may make you wary of seeing it as the last word on the matter.

Summary

Drawing on illustrative material from the changing constructions of and interventions towards people with mental health problems and people with learning difficulties, this section has shown that the medical model of disability is not itself unchanging or monolithic. However, the overriding message of this model has been seen by critics as that of the individualization of disability in terms of individual pathology (see Figure 2.1 overleaf). Furthermore, the model focuses on the impairment rather than the person, and power resides with the medical and allied professions. According to the orthodox medical discourse,

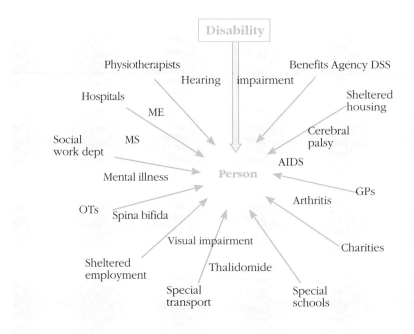

Figure 2.1 The medical model of disability

the explanation of the social problem of disability is based on a primary focus on the defective/impaired and thereby deviant characteristics of the individual body or mind which in turn is understood as vulnerable and dependent. As a clear illustration of the complex intertwining of social constructions and specific policy interventions, social and health policies have then been developed to deal with this apparently natural state of vulnerability and dependency.

It is arguably this medical and individualistic model which continues to inform most current policy interventions on disability. Thus even in anti-discrimination legislation such as the 1995 Disability Discrimination Act in Britain, disadvantage is seen in terms of the individual's impairment and lack of ability. As Priestley (1995, p.8) notes, this medical and individualistic paradigm of disability has led over the decades to a British social policy agenda in which there are 'disablement' services that deal exclusively with individual need and functional rehabilitation rather than collective needs and civil rights (of which more in section 6). As a result of the hegemony of this medical discourse over the meaning and nature of disability, it can be argued that most of us have inhabited a world in which disabled people have been seen and understood as a problem. As Abberley (1996, p.77) has noted, 'scientific' medical knowledge has been a crucial tool to reinforce and justify this exclusion.

By our use of the example of the medical discourse on disability, we have also introduced you to how appropriations of a given problem are realized in specific formations of power and knowledge. We have also seen that these formations are in turn embedded in concrete policies and practices in such institutions as the hospital and the school. Your further studies will show that similar issues exist within the discourses of other social issues/problems.

6   Disability as social oppression: the social model

We have already shown that what Chapter 1 referred to as 'hegemonic' constructions and their related definitions, practices and policies, such as we find in the individualized medical discourse of disability, have not gone unchallenged. Let us now look in some depth at the major challenge to the medical model of disability as presented by supporters of the social model of disability in the 1990s. This challenge can be said to have resulted in a new politics and a new emergent discourse on disability. However, since the 1980s it has been the activist disability movement that has been at the forefront of this new positioning in countries like the USA and the UK. Disabled activists have waged what may be termed 'language battles', 'rights campaigns' and 'identity wars' against the often collusive partners of the mass media, charities, medicine, law and the state in the oppression of disabled people. We will show that, as a result of such political struggles and new ways of theorizing associated with the social model of disability, new constructions of disability emerged which began to problematize the nature of 'able-bodiedness' itself.

6.1   The critique of the medicalization and individualization of disability

The social model of disability offers us a new 'paradigm' or conceptual framework for understanding disability in which it is not the physical, sensory, cognitive or mental impairment of the individual that disables, but rather disability results from the structural handicapping effects of a society geared towards able-bodiedness as the norm. This process is often termed 'disablement' by supporters of the social model. As a consequence, medicine, according to its critics, has played a key role in the process of naturalizing both able-bodiedness as 'health' and disability as 'individual sickness' or 'pathological condition'. In turn, the critique of the effects of the medicalization and individualization of the social problem of disability (as personal tragedy) has been a crucial starting point for the subsequent development of the social and structural model of disability as 'social oppression' (see Figure 2.2 overleaf).

social model

If we were to adopt the view that disability is a form of social oppression, how might this be translated into policies? It would perhaps lead to social policies which focused on disabled people as both the *collective* 'victim' and survivors of a prejudiced and discriminatory society rather than as *individual* victims of circumstance. Such social (rather than medical) policies would thus be geared to the alleviation of oppression rather than the compensation of individuals, and would lead to structural interventions such as the redistribution of resources, changing the physical environment, and equal rights policies (see Oliver, 1990, pp.2–3). According to the social model, a fixed notion of 'normality' would no longer be an ideal to aspire to. Thus trying to force people to walk when they are not capable of doing so without severe and often hidden costs would be considered inappropriate given the 'normal' use of mobility aids by non-disabled people in the shape of cars, planes, etc. As Morris (1991, p.10) notes, 'To put it simply, it is not the inability to walk which disables someone but the steps into the building.'

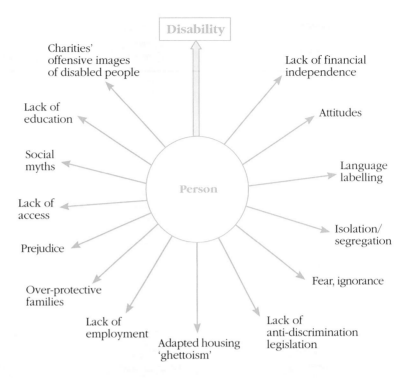

Disability

Charities'
offensive images
of disabled people

Lack of financial
independence

Lack of
education

Attitudes

Social
myths

Language
labelling

Person

Lack of
access

Isolation/
segregation

Prejudice

Fear, ignorance

Over-protective
families

Lack of
employment

Lack of
anti-discrimination
legislation

Adapted housing
'ghettoism'

Figure 2.2 The social model of disability: disabling forces at work

Let us briefly examine some of the criticisms of the medical definitions and interventions within disability.

In Extract 2.9, Michelle Mason recounts her childhood experiences of being photographed during a stay in hospital. Think about what the experience tells us about the status of the 'person' in medical regimes concerned with the diagnosis and classification of an impairment.

Extract 2.9 Mason: 'On the children's ward'

I remember too having medical photographs taken. I remember being told I was going to have some photographs taken and I thought, 'Oh, good!', thinking it was snapshots like my Dad used to take. And this man arriving with his equipment and cameras and things. I was in hospital and I was in the children's ward and they just put the screens round me and told me to take everything off. I couldn't understand and just did it. I didn't know what was happening from that point onwards, really. I just knew that he was taking bits, he wasn't taking me, he was taking bits of me. It was horrid. I thought it was really rude.

And I remember thinking what's he going to do with them, he'll put them in a book. And I think I asked him, I think I said, 'What's he going to do with them?', and I think he said, 'We're going to put them in a book'. And that's really all that I can remember. I was disgusted by it … I think it's a violation. It's an absolute violation of somebody's private being.

The knowledge that one's photograph is being used as an exhibit to be examined by total strangers is in itself a gross invasion of personal privacy. But, as if that were not bad enough, we are also required to perform live.

(Mason, in Sutherland, 1981, pp.122–3)

COMMENT

This account captures the routine invisibility of the person in terms of what Foucault (1972) has called 'the medical gaze'. It is also indicative of how procedures routinely carried out in the practices of the medical discourse 'transform' the nature of the subject, in this case a young girl in hospital. As a result of such medical procedures, the individual appears to be 'reified' or made into a thing-like object and reduced to a medical case, worthy of being visually recorded for her 'impaired body' alone. Mason appears to have experienced a process of 'dehumanization'.

■ ■ ■

Other critics of the medicalization of disability have noted that the medical emphasis on clinical diagnosis of the 'condition' tends to lead to a partial and inhibiting view of the disabled individual. Indeed, Brisenden (1986) contends that the problem of medicalization for the individual human being subjected to its discourse is particularly dangerous when the medical facts come to determine not only medication and treatment (if appropriate) but also the form of life for the person who happens to be disabled.

According to proponents of the social model of disability, a whole 'rehabilitation machine' has also built up around the hospital, itself predicated upon the institutionalization of the 'abnormality' of disabled people and the quest for future 'steps' towards approximate 'normality'.

Finkelstein, drawing on his own experience, analyses the process of rehabilitation as follows:

The aim of returning the individual to normality is the central foundation stone upon which the whole rehabilitation machine is constructed. If, as happened to me following my spinal injury, the disability cannot be cured, normative assumptions are not abandoned. On the contrary, they are re-formulated so that they not only dominate the treatment phase searching for a cure but also totally colour the helper's perception of the rest of that person's life. The rehabilitation aim now becomes to assist the individual to be as 'normal as possible'.

The result, for me, was endless soul-destroying hours at Stoke Mandeville Hospital trying to approximate to able-bodied standards by 'walking' with callipers and crutches ... Rehabilitation philosophy emphasises physical normality and, with this, the attainment of skills that allow the individual to approximate as closely as possible to able-bodied behaviour (e.g. only using a wheelchair as a last resort, rather than seeing it as a disabled person's mobility aid like a pair of shoes is an able-bodied person's mobility aid).

(Finkelstein, 1985, pp.4–5)

Through such analyses, proponents of the social model of disability alert us to the complex historical interplay of constructions, interventions and policy outcomes in the welfare state around the contested phenomenon of disability, the process of disablement and the ideology of disablism. The term 'disablism' **disablism** was first used by the disability movement to describe ideological processes (including medical knowledge) which legitimate the existing power structure based on discrimination and prejudice against disabled people.

This chapter, and those following on 'race' and sexuality, all argue strongly that words count. It is a well-established sociological adage that if people define situations as real, then they are real in their consequences. Thus if disability is defined and seen as a tragedy and/or a 'natural' and determining condition (as seems to have been the dominant categorization of disability in the UK in the twentieth century), then disabled people will be treated and responded to as if they are victims of a tragic accident or circumstance. In turn, the treatment is not just evident in routine day-to-day encounters and interaction, but will be translated into medical/rehabilitative policies that will aim to compensate – or even 'cure' – the tragic victims. Furthermore, the 'subjects' of such practices are in part 'constituted' through the interplay of representations, experiences and, perhaps more crucially, 'knowledges'.

6.2   The politics of the disability movement

Since the 1980s the disability movement in the UK, based on organizations of disabled persons, has been actively engaged in struggles to transform the political agenda for disabled people, reflected in the call for a shift from 'charity to rights' (Campbell and Oliver, 1996). A new 'rights discourse' has led to the possibility of an emergent construction of disabled people as socially, politically and legally oppressed citizens rather than dependent and needy individuals. In particular, we may note the concrete struggles both to change the law and use law to overcome discrimination in areas of social policy, such as employment, welfare rights and housing (Gooding, 1994). These struggles have been organized around what sociologists term the 'new social movement' of disability activists. Scott (1990, p.6) has argued that: 'A social movement is a collective actor constituted by individuals who understand themselves to have common interests and, for at least some significant part of their social existence, a common identity.' Furthermore, the defining characteristics of the new social movements (such as feminism and the ecology and disability movements) is their ability to rally and mobilize mass support around issues which cut across traditional divides (particularly those of class, nation and 'race').

Activists in the disability movement have sought to question the dominant construction of disability = dependency. For example, Oliver (1990) has noted that the logical opposite of dependency is no assistance from anyone. However, 'mutual interdependence' is a reality for all humans. The challenges to the dominant 'dependency' constructions described above are further consolidated by the significance and meaning given to the word 'independence' in the new discourse of the disability movement in the UK today. In this emergent 'expert' and politicized discourse, drawing heavily on the first-hand 'experienced' nature of disability, independence is thus defined in terms of people having control over their lives. As Brisenden (1986, p.140) notes, 'Independence is not linked to the physical or intellectual capacity to care for oneself without assistance; independence is created by having assistance when and how one requires it, by being able to choose when and how care takes place.' According to this alternative construction, independence or personal autonomy is about controlling one's own life, and that personal independence may in turn be facilitated through another body (Campbell and Oliver, 1996).

Perhaps not surprisingly, the struggle against residential/institutionalized care has been at the centre of the disability movement's political agenda and its fight for human rights for disabled people. This is evident in the following statement by the Union of the Physically Impaired Against Segregation (UPIAS):

> The reality of our position as an oppressed group can be seen most clearly in segregated residential institutions, the ultimate human scrap-heaps of the society. Thousands of people are sentenced to these prisons for life – which may these days be a long one. For the vast majority there is no alternative, no appeal, no remission of sentence for good behaviour, no escape except from life itself.
>
> (Union of Physically Impaired Against Segregation, 1981, p.2)

How does this statement 'politicize' the dominant form of institutional treatment which disabled people have historically received?

The quote challenges the dominant professional and state bureaucratic notions of residential, segregative care for disabled people as being 'in their best interests' and as operating as benevolent and therapeutic havens. The UPIAS statement employs the imagery of the prison and enforced incarceration in its critique of segregated residential institutions; indeed, the latter have, as institutions, shared a common ancestry with that of the prison (Foucault, 1977). Implicit in this statement is the support for 'independent' living in the community for all people who have physical, sensory, cognitive or mental impairments. Furthermore, the political agenda of the disability movement comprises civil rights, equal opportunities and independence rather than compensation, charity and pity. The chosen strategy in the 1990s has been that of confrontation and demand, with rights to be struggled for and won rather than given.

In the UK context, the disabled feminist writer Jenny Morris has argued that her own involvement in disability politics is 'driven by the anger and hurt I experience as a result of prejudice and discrimination … [and a] tremendous sense of powerfulness … [but is] also a celebration of our strength and a part of our taking pride in ourselves, a pride which incorporates our disability and values it' (Morris, 1991, p.14).

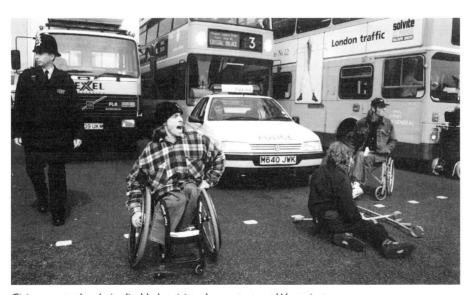

Giving way to the chair: disabled activists demonstrate at Westminster

Read the quote below from Jenny Morris on the rise of the 'disability culture' and re-read Extract 2.5 by Pam Evans on day-to-day experiences of disability in Activity 2.1.

Physical disability and illness are an important part of human experience. The non-disabled world may wish to try and ignore this and to react to physical difference by treating us as if we are not quite human, but we assert that our difference is both an essential part of human experience and, given the chance, can create important and different ways of looking at things.

(Morris, 1991, p.38)

What major challenges do these extracts raise for the constructions of disability discussed in sections 2, 4 and 5 of this chapter?

In sections 2, 4 and 5 above, the dominant images of disability have historically constituted disabled people as 'the other' and as lesser human beings, both distinct and inferior to the 'norm' of the able-bodied. In contrast to such inferiorization and separation of disabled people from non-disabled subjects, Morris's comments on the rise of a disability culture show the significance of disability to the lives and experiences of all humans. In a real sense, then, all humans are temporarily able-bodied, with phases of dependency and disablement whether due to the ageing process or periods of illness, injury, etc. The writings of Morris, Evans and others thus challenge the 'myth' of a sharp dichotomy between the 'disabled' and the 'able-bodied' and open up the possibility of new knowledges about human 'embodiment'. At the same time, the quotes by Morris and Evans also confirm the importance of 'difference' to an understanding of the lives of disabled people, like those of other oppressed groups in our society. Indeed, for Morris it is important to recognize difference in terms of the intellectual and physical characteristics of people, and that these characteristics often do imply additional needs, such as resources to live independently.

■ ■ ■

Writers such as Oliver (1990) confirm that the 'difference' experienced by disabled people is constituted by the processes of marginalization and oppression in society. Disabled people are therefore subject to a particular form of compounded oppression where they are both marginalized and discriminated against by social institutions and the able-bodied, and in turn this is compounded by the creation of dependency by welfare professionals. The specific demands of disabled people are thus about not just rights to employment and equal opportunities, but also control over and rights to welfare provision (Oliver, 1990, p.71). The politics of the disability movement has involved complex negotiations and struggles with the law, given the latter's great power as a form of knowledge which defines authoritatively what is 'normal'. Indeed, it has been argued that the law has been complicit in and vital to the historical hegemony of the medical discourse over disability (Gooding, 1994). However, the late twentieth-century struggles of the disability movement in the UK show that the law may also be a positive agent for social change and 'a forum for articulating alternative visions and accounts' (Smart, 1989, p.88).

The disability movement also sought to counter the dominant negative cultural imagery in the media and arts. This feature of new social movements

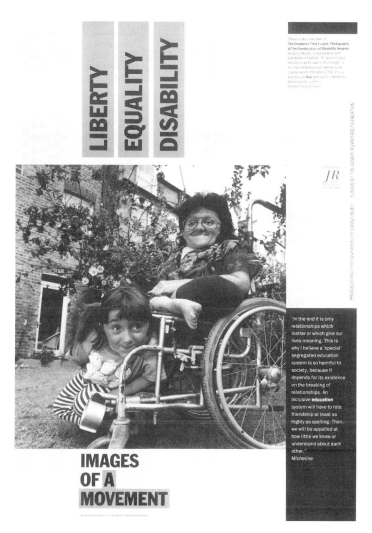

A campaign poster from the disability movement

has been described as 'identity wars'. Thus we may note the work of photographers such as Hevey (1992) in countering the charity representations discussed in section 4 above. In particular, Hevey and others have sought to challenge traditional representations and celebrate disabled people in terms of their profoundly 'energized bodies' and their human differences and similarities.

Other positive representations and thus what might be termed 're-constructions' of disabled people in the 1980s and 1990s were associated with the burgeoning literary trend within the disability movement: personal accounts, autobiographies, poems and such like sought to reclaim cultural spaces previously filled by negative stereotypes which we noted in section 2. The significance of such a new politics of identity should not be underestimated when we remember that representations become reproduced and 'solidified' as types of persons or subjects. Images have real effects for how people can live and what spaces are opened up or closed down. In turn, if disability is understood as a socially created construction, its meaning may be altered by social and political action (Gooding, 1994, p.26). Furthermore, identities are constructed in multiple and contradictory ways. As Barton (1996, p.11) has noted, disabled people are in a struggle to capture the power of naming 'difference' itself. The following poem by Lois Keith is one example of the challenges which disabled artists pose for dominant and taken-for-granted assumptions about the world:

Tomorrow I am going to re-write the English language

Tomorrow I am going to re-write the English language
I will discard all those striving ambulist metaphors
Of power and success
And construct new images to describe my strength
My new, different strength.
Then I won't have to feel dependent
Because I can't Stand On My Own Two Feet
And I will refuse to feel a failure
Because I didn't Stay One Step Ahead.
I won't feel inadequate
When I don't Stand Up For Myself
Or illogical because I cannot
Just Take It One Step at a Time
I will make them understand that it is a very male way
To describe the world
All this Walking Tall
And Making Great Strides.
Yes, tomorrow I am going to re-write the English Language,
Creating the world in my own image.
Mine will be a gentler, more womanly way
To describe my progress.
I will wheel, cover and encircle.
Somehow I will learn to say it all.

(Keith, 1994, p.57)

6.3   The unfinished and contested nature of the social model

The model of disability as 'social oppression' has itself been subject to criticism, confirming again that all constructions of social problems are subject to contestation. Let us look briefly at this debate. Mike Bury, a medical sociologist, has expressed 'academic' concerns about what he terms the 'politically correct' view of disability associated with the disability movement's work (Bury, 1996). According to Bury, much of the 'qualitative' work of the disability movement described above runs the risk of privileging personal 'experience' as a way of knowing over any sociological research methodology. Bury also noted that disabled researchers have raised ethical questions regarding the right of 'able-bodied' researchers to tackle issues to do with the politics of disability, since such researchers, as 'able-bodied', are necessarily part of the oppressive majority over the 'disabled' minority. In his critique of the work of some disabled researchers/activists, Bury notes that the complex relationship of chronic illness to disability is often not addressed in the radical disability movement literature. In Bury's view, most chronic medical conditions (which are largely found in older people) cause some degree of disability (defined by Bury in terms of restriction of activity or capacity for self-care). But, on the other hand, not all forms of disability (particularly those characteristic of many younger disabled people, resulting in Bury's terms from a congenital factor or traumatic injury) are either due to or involve chronic illness. Bury argues that 'social oppression' theory thus tends to act as an ideological underpinning of the activities of younger (mostly middle-class) people with the latter kind of non-chronic, relatively stable though perhaps severe forms of disability. To the extent that older people are affected by disabling chronic medical conditions, Bury contends that their interests may be poorly served by such ideas as 'disability is a form of social oppression', since the disability associated with older people often does require institutional and specialist social and medical care. Indeed, Bury argues that researchers need to defend and improve the medical and rehabilitative care (threatened in the health care reforms in the 1990s) for the 'voiceless' elderly disabled population. Bury suggests such support may in fact be undermined if the radical disability movement's campaigning were to focus public attention on those with the most developed voice who attack such care. In Bury's view, many old people living with chronic illnesses, at a time when the welfare state has been under attack, do not carry political weight in either mainstream politics or radical disability politics.

As an example of the systematic scepticism of social science to which you were alerted in Chapter 1, this critique is important in addressing the problem that the 'disabled' population is segmented and should not be treated as one conceptual category. The construction of disability by proponents of the 'social oppression' thesis and the independent living movement is thus, in the eyes of some critics, itself a selective representation of reality, arising out of a sectional rather than unified movement.

Not unexpectedly, there have been counter-arguments to Bury's critique. Oliver (1990, p.iv), for example, has contended that 'All disabled people experience disability as social restriction', and this would of course include older people with chronic illnesses. Barnes (1996) reaffirms the important point that, historically, academic research has been part of the oppression of disabled people, and the latter should be wary of the 'independent' researcher. Barnes goes on to question what he terms 'the myth of the independent researcher' and instead puts forward the following agenda for researchers: 'Researchers should be espousing commitment not value-freedom, engagement not objectivity, and solidarity not independence. There is no independent haven or middle ground when researching oppression: academics and researchers can only be with the oppressors or with the oppressed' (Barnes, 1996, p.110).

There have also been challenges to and contestation of the external 'social oppression' thesis and the profound 'social constructionist' view of the problems of disabled people from members of the disability movement itself. Thus Morris (1991) notes that the disability movement has been dominated by men and has tended to ignore and deny different experiences among categories of disabled people (just as she notes that 'able-bodied' feminists have denied different experiences and needs with regard to disabled women). According to Morris, the 'social model' has shown a tendency to deny the experience which disabled people have of their own bodies, insisting that physical differences and restrictions are entirely socially created. Morris accepts that environmental barriers and social attitudes are a crucial part of the experience of disability and that they do 'dis-able', but states that this is not 'all there is to it'. For Morris (1991, p.10), it is also vital not to deny personal experiences of physical/intellectual restraint, of illness, of the fear of dying.

Other challenges to the disability movement's attempt to construct a unified 'voice' for all disabled people emerged from groups defined traditionally as disabled, such as some activists among deaf people. Commenting on the misgivings of some deaf people on being called disabled, Davies (1993, p.6) notes: 'They conceive their own community as being separate from hearing society because of linguistic traditions. Deaf culture is based on the nurturing of a distinct language – British Sign Language, and therefore they perceive themselves as being a linguistic minority within society'. This argument for an autonomous deaf culture in the UK in the late twentieth century is perhaps most important for our purposes here in showing that the radical politics of the disability movement, and thereby its constructions of disability, are themselves 'contested'. In turn, Davies (1993, p.6) re-asserts the 'dominant' disability movement's ideological position on deaf people when he notes: 'Precisely because society does not recognize and endorse deaf people's language and needs, means that deaf people are disabled by society as much as the rest of the disabled community'.

Summary

As you will now be aware, the social model of disability questions the dominant construction of disability associated with the medical discourse and the charity/welfare state providers. It does so on a number of fronts in terms of its emphasis on disability being the result of legal discrimination and social oppression rather than an unfortunate 'condition' that some people possess. A new language of rights is thus opened up, and with it very different social policy agendas compared to the old welfare state dependency model of disability. We have also examined how the social model of disability 'reconstructs' the identities of disabled people through a variety of challenges to the dominant stereotypes of the 'disabled identity'. Furthermore, we have seen that the social model of disability has itself become embedded in the discourse of the disability movement and is 'unfinished' and subject to contestation. Overall, the social model of disability driven by disability movements in countries like the UK may offer us the possibility of a new discourse on the disability/able-bodiedness spectrum.

7   Conclusion

This chapter has explored the way in which the method of social constructionism may be illustrated through looking at 'disability'. Let us for the moment pretend that this has been a chapter about disability rather social constructionism. What have we learnt about disability? We have learnt the extent to which 'disability' can be best understood not as a natural/unnatural and unitary 'condition', but rather as a phenomenon subject to competing constructions. In the process we have revealed the complexities involved in what is understood to be 'disability'. Indeed, part of the problem of unearthing what is the reality of 'disability' has been the historical and cultural baggage associated with the concept itself. Historically the concept of disability has implied a unity to what is a vast array of experiences, practices and 'conditions'. Instead this chapter has argued that disability is necessarily an elusive category which needs to be subjected by social science to 'deconstruction'. It would seem that disability only comes alive through the meanings attached to it in specific socio-historical settings and through the different voices which speak its name.

This chapter has also been concerned with the interconnections between the social constructions of social problems and the nature of social interventions (including non-intervention) aimed at remedying or managing social problems. On the basis of the ground covered in this chapter it should be evident that the links between the definition of disability as a moral/medical/social problem and the appropriate form of intervention are both complex and specific and yet also comparable to other social problems. As a result this chapter has sought to offer the means of a critical deconstruction of an apparently simple concept and 'natural' state of being ('disability') which remains the site of political, medical, academic, legal and moral contestations. The contestation between the 'natural' and the 'social' has predominantly taken the form of the medical versus the social model of disability.

We shall end by summarizing what we have learnt about social construction from this chapter:

- It should be clear that images and stereotypes of social problems and 'deviant' populations are unlikely to be coherent or logical wholes but rather are often contradictory combinations of elements made up of different ideological 'traces'. This lesson has emerged from the tale we have told about the complex coalescence of moral, scientific and political notions of 'disability', but it would be equally pertinent to the study of, say, 'crime' or 'poverty'.

- We identified the significance of the normal = natural equivalence both in its own right and as a precondition for the existence of more specific discourses about the 'abnormal' and how to handle them. We examined this equivalence between the normal and the natural around religious, medical and welfarist representations of, and interventions towards, disabled people, but a similar argument could have been made with reference, for example, to the historical debates about homosexuality and 'impurity' (see Chapter 4).

- We have explored the crucial relationship between constructions and discourses. In particular, using the example of the medical discourse on disability, we have seen how systematic appropriations of the problem are realized in formations of power and knowledge and are embedded in what the sociologists Berger and Luckman (1967) famously termed 'institutionalized practices'. In more concrete terms, we have seen how the medical model, together with its variants, is a clear example of a discourse which 'owns' a problem.

- This chapter has plotted the growth of an increasingly influential 'social model' around one particular social problem, albeit it in the context of a still dominant medical discourse. Once again there are clear parallels to be drawn with contemporary debates around the issues of 'race' and sexuality which are explored further in Chapters 3 and 4.

- Finally, we have shown that social constructions have a solidity in everyday life which cannot be ignored and are real in their consequences for people.

Further reading

Since the early 1990s there has been a growing and increasingly influential body of literature written by activists in the disability movement. Campbell and Oliver (1996) offer an important introduction to the history of the disability movement in the UK.

Morris (1991) makes a vital contribution to the important debate around disability, gender and ethnicity.

Oliver (1990) remains the best introduction to the sociological understanding of disability. Barton (1996) adds to Oliver's sociological introduction with a collection of very readable and critical essays.

The history of disabled people's lives remains largely unwritten. However, Humphries and Gordon (1992) provide us with a compelling and very moving oral history of disabled people in Britain.

Hevey (1992) has produced an important text which challenges, partly through visual imagery, the dominant negative portrayal of disabled people in contemporary Britain and offers us new and important positive imagery of disabled people.

On the important changes in policy and practice around disability issues, see Bornat *et al.* (1993) and Swain *et al.* (1993). You are also recommended to look at the journal *Disability and Society* for specialist papers on this topic.

References

Abberley, P. (1996) 'Work, utopia and impairment', in Barton, L. (ed.) *Disability and Society*, London, Longman.

Arlidge, J. T. (1859) *On the State of Lunacy and the Legal Provision for the Insane*, London.

Bannister, D. (1981) 'Constructing a disability', in Brechin, A. *et al.* (eds) *Handicap in a Social World*, London, Hodder and Stoughton.

Barnes, C. (1992) *Disabling Imagery and the Media*, London, Ryburn Press.

Barnes, C. (1996) 'Disability and the myth of the independent researcher', *Disability and Society*, vol.11, no.1, pp.107–11.

Barton, L. (ed.) (1996) *Disability and Society: Emerging Issues and Insights*, London, Longman.

Berger, P. and Luckman T. (1967) *The Social Construction of Reality*, London, Allen Lane.

Bornat, J. *et al.* (eds) (1993) *Community Care*, Basingstoke, Macmillan.

Brisenden, S. (1986) 'Independent living and the medical model of disability', *Disability, Handicap and Society*, vol.1, no.2, pp.173–8.

Bruce, I. (1994) *Meeting Need: Successful Charity Marketing*, Hemel Hempstead, Institute of Chartered Secretaries and Administrators.

Burr, E. (1995) *Introduction to Social Constructionism*, London, Routledge.

Bury, M. (1996) 'Disability and the myth of the independent researcher: a reply', *Disability and Society*, vol.11, no.1, pp.111–15.

Campbell, J. and Oliver, M. (1996) *Disability Politics: Understanding Our Past, Changing Our Future*, London, Routledge.

Davidson, I. (1994) 'Images of disability in 19th century British children's literature', *Disability and Society*, vol.9, pp.33–45.

Davies, C. (1993) *Life Times: A Mutual Biography of Disabled People*, Farnham, Understanding Disability Educational Trust.

Department of Health and Social Security (1975) *Better Services for the Mentally Ill*, London, HMSO.

Dickens, C. (1843) *A Christmas Carol*, reprinted 1971 in *The Christmas Books*, vol.1, Harmondsworth, Penguin.

Douglas, M. (1966) *Purity and Danger*, London, Routledge.

Driedger, D. (1989) *The Last Civil Rights Movement*, London, HMSO.

Finkelstein, V. (1985) Paper given at WHO meeting, 24–28 June, Netherlands.

Foucault, M. (1971) *Madness and Civilization*, London, Tavistock.

Foucault, M. (1972) *The Archaeology of Knowledge*, New York, Harper and Row.

Foucault, M. (1977) *Discipline and Punish*, Harmondsworth, Penguin.

Freidson, E. (1970) *The Profession of Medicine*, New York, Dodd and Mead.

Fulcher, G. (1989) *Disabling Policies? A Comparative Approach to Education, Policy and Disability*, Lewes, Falmer.

Goffman E. (1961) *Asylums: Essays on the Social Situation of Mental Patients and Other Inmates*, Harmondsworth, Penguin.

Gooding, C. (1994) *Disabling Laws, Enabling Acts: Disability Rights in Britain and America*, London, Pluto.

Harrison, J. (1994) *Managing Charitable Investments*, Hemel Hempstead, Institute of Chartered Secretaries and Administrators.

Hattersley, J. (1987) *People with Mental Handicap*, London, Faber and Faber.

Hevey, D. (1992) *The Creatures Time Forgot*, London, Routledge.

Humphries, S. and Gordon, P. (1992) *Out of Sight: Experiences of Disability 1900–50*, Plymouth, Northcote.

Keith, L. (ed.) (1994) *Mustn't Grumble*, London, Women's Press.

Kurtz, R. (1981) 'The sociological approach to mental retardation', in Brechin, A. *et al.* (eds) *Handicap in a Social World*, London, Hodder and Stoughton.

Lonsdale, S. (1990) *Women and Disability*, London, Macmillan.

Miles, M. (1995) 'Disability in an eastern religious context: historical perspectives', *Disability and Society*, vol.10, no.1, pp.49–70.

Morris, J. (1991) *Pride Against Prejudice*, London, The Women's Press.

Oliver, M. (1990) *The Politics of Disability*, London, Macmillan.

Pearson, G. (1974) *The Deviant Imagination*, London, Macmillan.

Potts, P. (1982) 'Origins', Block 1 of E241 *Special Needs in Education*, Milton Keynes, The Open University.

Priestley, M. (1995) 'Dropping 'E's: the missing link in quality assurance for disabled people', *Critical Social Policy*, vol.15, no.2/3, pp.7–21.

Proctor, R. (1988) *Racial Hygiene: Medicine Under The Nazis*, Cambridge, MA., Harvard University Press.

Quicke, J. (1985) *Disability in Modern Children's Fiction*, London, Croom Helm.

Rieser, R. and Mason, M. (eds) (1990) *Disability Equality in the Classroom: A Human Rights Issue*, London, ILEA.

Scott, A. (1990) *Ideology and the New Social Movements*, London, Unwin Hyman.

Scull, A. (1979) *Museums of Madness: The Social Organization of Insanity in Nineteenth Century England*, New York, St Martin's Press.

Sedgwick, P. (1982) *Psychopolitics*, London, Pluto.

Shakespeare, T. (1995) 'Back to the future? New genetics and disabled people', *Critical Social Policy*, vol.15, no.2/3, pp.22–35.

Smart, C. (1989) *Feminism and the Power of the Law*, London, Routledge.

Stevenson, R.L. (1883) *Treasure Island*, reprinted 1983, Harmondsworth, Penguin.

Sutherland, A. (1981) *Disabled We Stand*, London, Souvenir.

Swain, J. *et al.* (eds) (1993) *Disabling Barriers, Enabling Environments*, London, Sage.

Thomas, K. (1971) *Religion and the Decline of Magic*, Harmondsworth, Penguin.

Topliss, E. (1982) *Social Responses to Handicap*, Harlow, Longman.

Townsend, P. (1967) *The Disabled in Society*, London, Greater London Association for the Disabled.

Tuke, S. (1813) *A Description of the Retreat at York*, reprinted 1964 as facsimile edition, edited by Hunter, B. and MacAlpine, I.

Union of Physically Impaired Against Segregation (UPIAS) (1981) Editorial in *Disability Challenge*, 1 May.

Warnock, M. (1978) *Special Educational Needs: The Report of the Committee of Enquiry into the Education of Handicapped Children and Young People*, London, HMSO.

Williams, F. (1992) 'Women with learning difficulties are women too', in Langan, M. and Day, L. (eds) *Women, Oppression and Social Work*, London, Routledge.

Wood Committee (1929) *Report of the Mental Deficiency Committee*, London, HMSO.

CHAPTER 3

Welfare and the Social Construction of 'Race'

by Gail Lewis

Contents

1   Introduction

This chapter will consider the links between the idea of 'race' and the development of a number of education policies and debates which occurred in England and Wales between the 1960s and the 1980s. It will focus on:

■   The ways in which a bundle of 'natural' material called 'the body' is given social meaning.

■   The way in which such social meanings give rise to policy debates and formulations which then reproduce or rework these social meanings.

Reference is made in the chapter to 'meanings attached to particular bodies' in order to help convey the way in which bodies are socially constructed and treated *as if* the owners of particular types of body have specific characteristics. The chapter does this principally by looking at how the idea of 'race' has influenced and been reflected in education policy and debate. But why is this relevant to a book whose focus of concern is the social construction of social difference and social problems? The answer can be found in the three main conceptual themes of the chapter. These are:

1   The distinction which social scientists make between essentialist and social constructionist perspectives as discussed in Chapter 1.

2   The process by which social relations are seen to be 'natural' relations and 'outside' of society – that is, the social is constructed as natural.

3   The ways in which public debate and social policy reflect particular conceptions of what is a 'social problem', and why it is one; and how they further define more general social meanings which affect everyday life – that is, the ways in which social policies construct social problems.

We aim to help you to develop your understanding of these themes by focusing here on the link between the idea of 'race' and education policy and debate.

'race'

If the argument of the chapter is that 'race' is a socially constructed category, why begin with the body? The answer is quite complex, but may be summed up in two points. The first is the apparently obvious: the visible physical variations to be found amongst the human population in terms of skin colour, average size, hair texture, eye and nose shape and so on – that is, those physical characteristics used to classify and group people into 'races'. In this sense, then, there is variation among human groups and it would silly to deny this.

To recognize such variation is not at all the same thing as saying that such variation gives rise to differences in intellectual, social or physical capabilities. We cannot read off from visible physical variation among humans a range of capabilities, desires or potentialities. At least, the social constructionist cannot; the essentialist, on the other hand, will start precisely with these differences. In contrast to the essentialist, however, the social constructionist will be interested in exploring the *meanings* attached to such physical variation – and this is the second reason for starting with the body.

social
constructionist

This chapter will use extensively the words 'race', ethnicity and nation(ality) – all words with which most of us are familiar. We hear them on radio and television, we read them in newspapers and magazines, we speak them in everyday conversations. But what do they refer to and how do they differ from each other? These are important considerations and social scientists writing within a social constructionist perspective are concerned with asking a series of such questions. For example:

- What is the context in which these terms are being used?

- Who is using them, and with what effects?

- What ideas about the state of relations between diverse groups in society is conveyed in any particular use of one or other of these terms?

- What senses of self and group belonging are conveyed by the use of them?

- Does the use of these terms by particular individuals and groups, in specific contexts, have any relevance?

By addressing such questions in this chapter, familiar words are cast in a new and different light, making apparently simple and self-evident terms difficult, and it is important to remember this as you read through the chapter – it requires the adoption of a sceptical stance towards much current understanding of these terms and that you think about how they are being used here.

2 Stories of bodies, 'race' and place: two women, two cities

The bodies that we occupy matter (Butler, 1993). The names given to our physical characteristics are one of the means by which we are categorized into 'types' of people. Predominant amongst those 'types' with which we are most familiar are the categories of woman, man, black, white, old, young, disabled, able-bodied, fat, thin, tall and short. Our bodies, or the names attached to them, are one of the ways in which our location in the world is marked. Alongside the categorization of people on the basis of their physical characteristics is the suggestion that particular characteristics also indicate *capabilities* – whether these be intellectual, physical or social. Thus our bodily characteristics are also given meaning and become the basis on which we 'read' them – as belonging to a particular group, having a certain status, being able to do certain things: even to go to or to move about in particular places.

meaning

ACTIVITY 3.1

Try to remember any occasions when you have been 'placed' in a certain way because of the body you have. Think about the characteristics which were being used to place you in this particular way, and briefly list them.

COMMENT

You may have thought of the common ideas that fat people are always jolly or dirty; that women are 'naturally' caring, men 'naturally' aggressive; that people of African origin or descent are 'naturally' good at athletics or boxing (if male) but unable to swim; that Jewish people are crafty, mean money grabbers; that Irish people are drunkards, violent and 'thick'; and that old people are decrepit and dependent. If you did find that you were thinking along these lines, it is because this is the 'common-sense' way (see Chapter 1) of thinking about physical variation. We assume that it is possible to tell what a person is like or able to do, on the basis of how they look. What a social constructionist perspective encourages is an exploration behind these assumptions to see how it is they arise and what their social implications might be.

■ ■ ■

Having a body, then, means not only having a specific genetic make-up but also having specific *social* locations. It is this last aspect on which we wish to concentrate in this chapter. There are two aspects to this. On the one hand, the physical characteristics of our bodies help to form our *identities* – that is, our sense of who we are and of those other people whom we assume are like us. This sense of self and group belonging suggests that the 'individual' is located in a wider network of people who share something in common – that is, who have a social identity, with an individual and collective history. On the other hand, the positions we occupy are also given to us, they are ascribed, and one of the mechanisms used for the ascription of a place within sets of social relations is the body. The meanings attached to physical characteristics highlight the *social* or *constructed* nature of our bodies. It is also through this ascription of meaning that we can begin to grasp the relationship between our bodies and the factors through which social relations are structured.

social identity

ACTIVITY 3.2

Read Extracts 3.1 and 3.2. As you do so, try to identify the factors that were being 'carried' in the bodies of the two speakers. Consider how 'race' was important. Were there also elements of class? Did gender matter? And what issues of 'space' were raised?

Extract 3.1 Bruce-Pratt: 'Skin, blood, heart'

I live in … Washington, DC … . When I walk the two-and-a-half blocks … to stop in at the bank, to leave my boots off at the shoe-repair-and-lock shop, I am most usually the only white person in sight. …

When I walk three blocks in a slightly different direction down Maryland Avenue, to go to my lover's house, I pass the yards of Black folks: the yard of the lady who keeps children, with its blue-and-red windmill, its roses-of-sharon; the yard of the man who delivers vegetables with its stacked slatted crates; the yard of the people next to the Righteous Branch Commandment Church-of-God (Seventh Day) with its tomatoes in the summer, its collards in the fall. In the summer, folks sit out on their porches or steps or sidewalks; when I walk by, if I lift my head and look toward them and speak, 'Hey', they may speak, say, 'Hey', or 'How you doing?' or perhaps just nod. In the spring, I was afraid to smile when I spoke, because that might be too familiar, but by the end of summer I had walked back and forth so often, I was familiar, so sometimes we shared comments about the mean weather.

I am comforted by any of these speakings for, to tell you the truth, they make me feel at home. I am living far from where I was born; it has been twenty years since I lived in that place where folks, Black and white, spoke to each other when they met on the street …

The pain, of course, is the other side of this speaking, and the sorrow: when I have only to turn two corners to go back in the basement door of my building, to meet Mr Boone, the janitor, who doesn't raise his eyes to mine, or his head, when we speak. He is a dark red-brown man … When we meet in the hall or on the elevator, even though I may have just heard him speaking in his own voice to another man, he 'yes ma'am's' me in a sing-song: I hear my voice replying in the horrid cheerful accents of a white lady: and I hate my white womanhood that drags between us the long bitter history of our region.

I think how I just want to feel at home, where people know me; instead I remember, when I meet Mr Boone, that home was a place of forced subservience, and I know that my wish is that of an adult wanting to stay a child: to be known by others, but to know nothing, to feel no responsibility.

Instead, when I walk out in my neighbourhood, each speaking to another person has become fraught, for me, with the history of race and sex and class; as I walk I have a constant interior discussion with myself, questioning how I acknowledge the presence of another, what I know or don't know about them and what it means how they acknowledge me. It is an exhausting process, this moving from the experience of the 'unknowing majority' (as Maya Angelou called it) into consciousness. It would be a lie to say this process is comforting.

(Bruce-Pratt, 1988, pp.323–4)

Extract 3.2 Lewis: 'From deepest Kilburn'

Granville Road was a long street running between Kilburn Park at one end and Queens Park at the other. On our side of the road it began with a pub at the corner, then the laundry and the baths which took up a good stretch. There were also some warehouses behind the laundry, the place where many of us girls received some initiation into the secrets of sexual play. For me such 'experimentation' was often quite a frightening event because the big boys were the same ones who were always calling me 'nigger' or 'sambo' or 'junglebunny'. My 'going with them' was out of both fear (they threatened us with all sorts of things if we didn't) and, in a funny sort of way, an attempt to fit in, to become one of the gang and get them to stop calling me names. It was only when I was in my twenties that it struck me that this was simply a continuation of the centuries-long relationship between white men/boys and black women/girls. …

The whole street was a patchwork of no-go and go areas for me. I was not allowed to go into the playground because that's where a lot of the young Teds [Teddy Boys] hung out; I couldn't go too far to the other end, nor was I supposed to play back and forth across the road, though I did. I was only allowed to cross the road to go to school, get things from the shops two streets away for Mum, and to go to the White Knight [laundry]. I could go to the Rec [recreation ground], but I wasn't to hang around in those parts of the street where people from the house couldn't see me and where the Teds hung out. Mum and Dad were frightened that racialist adults or children would abuse me or even physically harm me, particularly because I was a girl.

I negotiated this chequerboard of on-off bounds easily and didn't really experience it as hardship. The only thing to avoid was the gangs and individuals who were at great pains to keep 'their territory' free of 'blacks'. In fact another bit of the road, which we called 'Little Granville', was full of kids with this aim in mind. …

As it happens I can't actually remember any particular incident that demonstrated the need for observing the no-go divisions in the street. Which isn't to say that the fears of the adults existed only in their paranoic minds. Our house was in fact firebombed during the 1958 Notting Hill riots, fortunately with no particularly harmful material results. … The incident certainly gave meaning to the chequerboard, because it operated to keep my playing area carefully demarcated from the houses and hang-outs of any youths suspected of being sympathetic to the racists, or even those who looked like Teddy boys.

I did, however, have one other source of protection. That was my babysitter friend, Sheila. Sheila was a young girl who lived down the road from us; her family was very poor and because they liked us and needed the money they let Sheila be my babysitter. But because Sheila and her family had lived in the street for years and were white, I got a kind of extra protection because she knew me. Anyway, she could fight and threatened to beat up anybody who did anything to me. Sheila was my friend as well and it was she who would take me and collect me from Brownies on a Friday night, which was how I got to go in the first place.

(Lewis, 1985, pp.219–21)

COMMENT

The first of these extracts, by Minnie Bruce-Pratt, is about a white woman in the USA living in an area of Washington, DC, delineated as 'black'. As she takes us on her journey through the streets of her neighbourhood she shows us the ways in which social relations, structured or organized through 'race', have a geographical or spatial dimension. Over the months her initial fear about being in a black area begins to evaporate into comfort and, despite the 'racial difference', *home* is evoked for her. This is made possible because of the daily interactions with her neighbours which allow her to speak across the difference of 'race' – a situation which we are given to understand is not a common occurrence.

However, we soon see that this situation is not all it appears to be because such speaking is only possible in a very specific context in which the geography is not also loaded with a class relation. We get a sense of this because Bruce-Pratt contrasts the interactions between herself and black people on the street, with her interaction with the janitor (caretaker) of her building. Here the altered social location – now both 'race' and class – in turn alters the very *tone and bodily demeanour* of the interaction between herself and a black man. From this she experiences her body in a different way – a way made heavy with the *history* of 'race', gender and class relations in the USA.

This then forces her to reconsider her memory of 'home' as a *comfortable* place uninfluenced by the social relations carried by bodily differences. Instead, she is forced to recognize the *subservience* which *structured* interactions between people of different 'races' and which was echoed in her encounter with the janitor. The effect of this reorganized memory of home is that now all her movements in her neighbourhood are laden with an awareness of how the meanings and histories attached to gender, 'race' and class are always inflected in 'inter-racial' interaction – they are *never innocent* of personal and collective history.

In the second extract by Gail Lewis, we move to north-west London in the 1950s, and here it is black people living in a 'white' area. Again we are made aware of the ways in which geographies are laden with meanings attached to 'race' and gender, and again these meanings and histories influence how *space is negotiated*. We see that *'threat'* is carried by history, but threat can only be known via the *'racial' meanings* attached to space. The threat serves to structure behaviour but only sometimes does this spill over into actual violence – as in the events in Notting Hill. What we also see clearly in this second extract is that the meanings ascribed to and carried by bodies are often gleaned by the way the body is *adorned*. Thus 'even those who looked like Teddy boys' were understood as threatening – their dress carried the meaning. In this extract more substance is given to the possibility of speaking across 'racial' divides since a friendship, rather than a neighbourly interaction, is evoked in the reference to Sheila. But even this is not uncomplicated since it is also portrayed as being mediated by a monetary relationship.

■ ■ ■

There is, then, a sense in which our bodies can be understood as cultural artefacts which carry the traces of social relations and which also express these social relations. Turner (1996) has suggested that to view the body in this way means at least three things.

First there is the idea that viewing the body as a cultural artefact means that the physical potentialities of the body are only realized in a social context, which may give rise to particular body practices, as in, say, ways of walking. Thus, though the human body carries with it the potential for walking, the actual style of walking will vary across time, place and other social divisions such as gender. Think, for example, of ways of walking associated with being a young woman or man in the UK today.

A second sociological approach to the body is the conceptualization of the body as a system of signs – that is, bearers of meaning – such that bodies can be read for what they say about, for example, class, or 'race', or gender.

Third, this approach can be extended to link the system of meanings attached to the body to the relations of power which predominate in any time or place. Thus the categorization of groups of bodies into types of people is also connected to the *hierarchical* ordering of these categories into a series of overlapping dominant and subordinate identities and positions. Thus whether we are female or male, black or white, old or young, disabled or able-bodied will perhaps have greater social, as opposed to personal, significance than if we are classified as of 'normal' height, or blue-eyed or brown-eyed, because of the ways in which the former positions reflect power relations. We can see an example of this in Extracts 3.1 and 3.2. The two speakers' understanding of the historical and contemporary relations which were carried by their bodies, provided the frames through which they negotiated their movement through their home environments.

categorization

Summary

In this section we have focused on three main points. First, we have considered the ways in which particular physical features are interpreted and used to construct distinct social groups known as 'races' – that is, we have considered the naturalization of a social production. Second, by looking at Extracts 3.1 and 3.2, we have considered ways in which such interpretations provide a framework through which individuals, who are ascribed to racial categories, understand and give meaning to their experiences. Third, we were briefly introduced to some social scientific approaches to 'reading' the body and, in particular, to the links between the social meanings attached to physical variation and systems of power relations.

The last two approaches – those of investigating the meanings attached to bodies and the ways in which these meanings express the relations of power which underlie the social arrangements of any given society – are consistent with a social constructionist approach to the body. Like Chapters 2 and 4, this chapter is concerned with exploring the links between the meanings attached to certain aspects of the body. Here we are concerned with those characteristics which are known as *racial characteristics* and through which human beings are grouped into 'races'. More specifically we shall be looking at the ways in which racial categorization has been linked to the process of inclusion in and exclusion from aspects of welfare.

3   Bodies and social exclusions

If the meanings attached to bodies indicate some of the structures of inequality which characterize a given society, so too does the idea of social exclusion. At a most basic level, to be excluded from something means being denied access to an activity, a place, or a range of resources. Apart from accident or oversight, such denials of access can be the result either of failure to meet specified conditions of entry, or of lack of financial resources. As such, exclusions can be the result of both formal and informal, direct and indirect, rules or arrangements. For example, to be denied access to something because you do not have the money required for entry is the result of indirect arrangements. This is because it is linked to the distribution of financial resources among a set of individuals and groups rather than because of the imposition of a set of rules or conditions. But to say that this type of exclusion is informally produced is not the same thing as saying that it is not structurally produced – that is, that it results from the ways in which relations between groups of people who stand in unequal relation to each other are organized.

3.1   National belonging, class and social exclusion

It was precisely this type of structurally produced exclusion that concerned the writer T.H. Marshall. He was particularly concerned with the ways in which social class position was related to processes of exclusion in terms of 'the extent to which those without money are unable to use leisure facilities, join evening classes, participate in political activity' (Levitas, 1996). Centrally, it was the relationship between poverty and citizenship on which Marshall focused, but citizenship for him comprised more than just the legal status of being a national of a particular country. Marshall made a distinction between three aspects of citizenship rights, each of which was interrelated. These are:

1   The *civil aspect:* this concerns individual freedoms associated with the right to free speech, to religious observation, to own property or to enter into legal contracts. It has, then, a legal aspect to it in so far as the law in democratic states should protect individual freedoms.

2   The *political aspect:* this is concerned with the democratic rights of participation in the polity: 'By the political element I mean the right to participate in the exercise of political power, as a member of a body invested

with political authority or as an elector of the members of such a body' (Marshall, 1950, p.11). (Note that Marshall uses the term 'body' here to refer to an institution or agency.)

3   The *social aspect:* 'By the social element I mean the whole range from the right to a modicum of economic welfare and security to the right to share to the full in social heritage and to live the life of a civilized being, according to the standard prevailing in the society' (Marshall, 1950, p.11).

Issues of inequality have been central to notions of exclusion from citizenship in the fullest sense of the term and central to this has been the notion that there is a universal right to a minimum standard of life. In addition, this notion of citizenship has carried with it the idea that state power must be used to mediate the inequalities which derive from a capitalist organization of society by ensuring 'equality in the distribution and realization of citizenship rights' (Faist, 1995, p.14).

We have begun this section by looking at the ways in which social exclusion has been linked to the denial of citizenship rights which ensue from social class, particularly in relation to the unequal distribution of material resources which result in poverty. Class is, however, only one among a number of ways in which populations are fragmented into discrete social categories or groups. Chapters 2 and 4 suggest that disability and sexuality are two others, and we will look now at the way in which 'race' is a further means of fragmenting the population into social groups and organizing the social relations among them.

3.2   Some indications of 'racially' ordered exclusions from welfare

By now it should be clear that the term 'race' is used here to refer to the construction of a category of belonging on the basis of physical variations found among human bodies. That is, it is being used to refer to a *social construction* and not a biologically given 'fact'.

ACTIVITY 3.3

Think over what you have read so far and list the key words which indicate the social constructionist approach to 'race' adopted here.

COMMENT

You may have included some of the following in your list of key words: categorization; meaning; experience; and social power.

From a social constructionist perspective what is important is the ways in which these terms link together to produce a *social relation* which organizes how people are placed in society. From this viewpoint, to construct groups of people into 'races' involves a threefold process:

1   Human populations are divided into discrete categories on the basis of variations in physical features.

2   Meaning is ascribed to this physical variation and it is then said to be possible to know the potentialities, behaviours, needs and abilities of a person on the basis of their 'racial' belonging.

3 This *social* process of categorization and classification is then said to be a product of nature – that is, racial division is said to be natural

natural

racialization   This process is often referred to as a process of racialization

■ ■ ■

Colour coding or description?

The categorization of human populations into 'races' is also a means of constructing borders or boundaries between social groups. One of the most obvious and common ways to see the link between the construction of both 'races' and borders is in terms of an entity called 'the nation'.

Benedict Anderson (1983) has suggested that 'the nation' is not a 'real' grouping but rather an 'imagined community' in which imaginary ties of a common ancestry and a common history are the means by which a sense of belonging is achieved. They are *imagined* ties because any individual member of a 'nation' will only ever meet or interact with a tiny minority of all those who are said to be of the same nation. It is imagined as *community* because, despite profound inequalities, 'the nation' is 'conceived as a deep, horizontal comradeship' (Anderson, 1983, p.6). But of course it is also a means of constructing a border or boundary between 'us' and 'them'.

nation

Nations tend to be imagined as racially and ethnically homogeneous and therefore Anderson's approach is useful for our purposes because it helps us to think about the links between the body and the nation. Remember that both are to be understood as social constructs – bodies, or physical variations among bodies, are given meaning as a result of which categories of belonging emerge. In this approach bodily 'features' – especially, but not only, colour – can be read as a means of identifying who automatically and 'rightfully' belongs within the border of the nation. If the nation is imagined as being made up of people said to be the same colour and said to have the same ethnic origins, then all those who are defined as not meeting these two criteria can be constructed as being 'outside' the nation, as not rightfully a part of it. So 'race' can be mapped on to 'the nation' to produce a structure for excluding groups of people either from entering the borders of the nation at all, or, if 'inside', from having access to the full range of 'economic welfare and security … [and] social heritage' which Marshall (1950, p.11) identified. This may be understood by thinking about the link between the structure and rules of immigration control and welfare benefits and services. There are three important points to note at the outset.

First, the exclusion of racialized groups from access to welfare benefits and/ or services goes back at least to the 1905 Aliens Act. This Act was passed to control entry into the UK of Jewish people fleeing persecution in Eastern Europe. Such potential migrants were defined as 'undesirable aliens', who should be excluded, if they were 'lunatics, persons of notoriously bad character or likely to become a charge upon public funds' (Bevan, 1986, p.69).

Second, since the 1960s, the treatment of black people in the UK, especially if they are poor, has been framed by a series of immigration and nationality laws and rules. These have had the effect of withdrawing or restricting the rights of black Commonwealth citizens (and their descendants). The 1962 Immigration Act began the process by restricting the right of entry of British citizens from the New Commonwealth and Pakistan. These citizens were only allowed in for primary immigration purposes if they could secure a work voucher. In the 1971 Immigration Act entry for such people was determined by the ability to prove a traceable link to a British grandparent or parent – known as the patriality clause. This process has continued:

> The 1981 Nationality Act removed the right to British citizenship by virtue of birth on British soil and deprived Commonwealth citizens settled here since 1973 of their automatic right to register as British citizens … the 1988 Immigration Act abolished the right of British and long-settled Commonwealth citizen men to be joined by their wives and children.
> (Lister, 1990, p.53)

Third, the exclusions on the basis of 'racial' categorization are not separate from the exclusions associated with class. That is, 'race' and class will often overlap so that members of racialized groups who are also economically poor will experience more disadvantage in relation to welfare than those amongst the middle or upper classes. For example, many people who are subject to immigration control, but who also require the assistance of welfare benefits or services, are sometimes denied access to these services and benefits because they are also subject to a condition where they must have 'no recourse to public funds'. In the UK in the late twentieth century immigration authorities have defined public funds as income support, family credit, housing benefit and housing provided by public bodies (Gurney, 1993).

Legislation has, then, progressively altered the terms on which black people from the Commonwealth can gain legal citizenship and this has had the knock-on effect of excluding people from access to welfare services and benefits. Moreover, the requirement not to have 'recourse to public funds' often acts as a means of internal control because it is linked to the association between 'race' and citizenship:

> In 1980, Lulu Bann, a commissioner of the Commission for Racial Equality who had lived in the UK for 14 years, was asked to produce her passport before she was admitted to a hospital in South London. The hospital refused to accept her doctor's letter and the fact that she had previously been treated at the hospital as proof that she was entitled to free treatment. ...
>
> In 1979, it was reported that a Cypriot woman had gone to a London hospital for an appointment with a surgeon. A hospital clerk, suspicious of the woman's immigration status, checked with the Department of Health and Social Services which, in turn, checked with the Home Office. It was discovered that the woman's appeal against deportation had been refused. The clerk then informed the Department of the woman's home address and the date of her next appointment.
>
> (Gordon and Klug, 1985, pp.19, 20)

This illustrates two points:

1   Exclusions from legal citizenship give rise to exclusions from social citizenship in the sense laid out by Marshall.

2   In this context, bodily features which are used to categorize people into 'races' may have the effect of obscuring the distinctions of legal citizenship and status among people defined as belonging to the same 'racial' category. In other words, the visibility of colour or other markers of 'racial difference' may have the effect of making other differences invisible.

Thus there is a variety of ways in which social exclusion occurs. For this reason some writers have argued that the idea of exclusion linked to Marshall's conception of citizenship (especially in its social aspect) must be broadened to take on board other statuses and positions, such as being a woman, a child or a member of an 'ethnic minority'. As Hall and Held have put it:

> A contemporary 'politics of citizenship' must take into account the role the social movements have played in *expanding* the claims to rights and entitlements to new areas. It must address not only the issues of class and inequality, but also questions of membership posed by feminism, the black and ethnic movements, ecology ... and vulnerable minorities like children.
>
> (Hall and Held, 1989, p.17)

And, as Chapter 2 points out, the disabled people's movement raises similar concerns.

These writers are pointing to a recognition that social exclusion from the full range of activities, enjoyments, rights and duties, which are part of full citizenship, results not just from a person's position in the class hierarchy but also from other social positions. We would call these 'subordinated positions' because, in comparison with men, those not defined in terms of an ethnicity, or as adults, those people defined as women or 'ethnic minorities' or children are denied full access to social citizenship. The exclusions which result from these positions are effected in different ways to those of social class. When we talk of the exclusions which emerge from social class, we are referring principally to economic relations. When we talk of gender, however, or of ethnicity or age, we are referring to other sets of relations organized around differences which are said to emerge from physical variation (that is, bodies) and the meanings and roles which are attached to this.

ACTIVITY 3.4

Think about the meanings and roles attached to being a man or a woman. How might they lead to reduced access to social citizenship rights for women? Make a note of your response before reading on.

COMMENT

When I thought about this I began with the sexual division of labour in households and paid employment. For example, in many heterosexual households women are defined as being dependent on men financially and emotionally. They tend to have prime responsibility for the care of children and other dependent relatives, and for the housework and cooking, all of which are unpaid duties – in fact, in official statistics and documents they are not defined as work at all. Where women do engage in paid employment they tend to be concentrated into particular occupations and industries – those areas defined as 'women's work' – and they tend to earn less than men. All these factors result in many women being financially dependent upon men and having to juggle domestic and employment responsibilities. They are then denied access to full participation in the range of activities associated with full citizenship, as identified by Marshall, because of financial and time constraints.

■ ■ ■

In addition to the exclusions which arise from structural arrangements there are also exclusions which result from the ways in which things are described and seen. For example, if a particular nation of people is always referred to in a way which suggests that these people are all of one ethnicity or 'race', though it is actually composed of a diverse mix of 'races' and ethnicities, then there will be exclusions. These exclusions are produced through processes of representation **representation** – that is, through the chains of meanings and associations which are attached to particular places, events, acts or people. We have already seen examples of this in Extracts 3.1 and 3.2. What was also evident from these extracts was that the experience of space, as organized through divisions of 'race', gender and class, was only possible because the meanings were collectively shared and understood by all those with whom the women interacted. That is, the spaces were *cultural* and acted as the starting-points for interactions across the 'racial' divides.

Summary

In this section you have been introduced to:

- The idea that social exclusion has been seen as mainly being derived from class.
- The reasons why some people have challenged this narrow approach to social exclusion.
- The distinctions and links between legal and social citizenship.
- The link between the idea of 'race' and that of the nation.
- The distinction between structural location and representation.
- The idea that social constructions have material effects in that they position people in social relations – they produce subjects or 'types' of people – and that these are reflected in policies and practices which lead to the reproduction of the constructions.

In the following sections we will consider further the social exclusions which emerge as a result of 'race' and ethnicity. The focus will be on education but it is important to remember that this is not a chapter *about* education. Rather, we use education as a site of policy in order to illustrate the social construction of social difference.

4   Education

One place to begin looking at the complex interweaving of exclusions and inclusions is in the field of education in England and Wales. This is an appropriate place to start since it is education that has the longest history of policy response and practice in relation to black people since the Second World War. The British population has a centuries-long history of diverse ethnic groups as successive waves of people from various parts of the globe came and settled here either as migrants or as conquerors (see, for example, Fryer, 1984; Kearney, 1995). **Hickman (1998)** has noted that a link between ethnic diversity and the construction of social problems was a feature of state education policy in nineteenth-century Britain. We can see a similar association being made in the wake of the post-Second World War migration and settlement of people from the Caribbean and the Indian sub-continent. It was generally agreed that this presence was understood as a problem (Mullard, 1982; Department of Education and Science, 1985) about which speedy action needed to be taken. In the process 'Black minorities have frequently been casualties of rules and procedures which may not have been intended to discriminate against them but which in effect, do so and there is considerable resistance when hitherto taken-for-granted procedures are brought into question' (Rattansi, 1992, p.23).

Much has been written about this history, but for our purposes we will organize the discussion around the ways in which the policy responses in education acted to exclude black pupils from images of the nation, and the 'normal' school population, despite the fact that the stated aims of these policies was precisely the opposite: that is, they were designed to facilitate inclusion. In reviewing this process we will consider the different policy 'moments' as they unfolded and the distinctions and similarities between them. Remember that we are using education as a means to explore the ways in which boundaries of exclusion and inclusion have been constructed around notions of 'race', ethnicity, culture and nation. In looking at the trajectories taken in education policy, therefore, our concern will be the social meanings attached to the presence of black pupils in schools up and down the country, which were carried by particular policy phases.

4.1 The development of policy

The starting-point for the emergence of education policy aimed at responding to the presence of black pupils in schools was that these pupils were viewed as a problem to be solved as quickly as possible. Mullard (1982) has suggested that the 'problem' was seen to reside in differences of colour, culture and language. The official response therefore necessitated both administrative and political dimensions. This understanding of the issues remained a dominant one right up to the late 1990s despite shifts in policy approaches and in underlying political approaches – both inside and outside central and local government. Up until the late 1980s it is possible to characterize these developments in policy orientation as having their *assimilationist* phase, their *integrationist* phase and their *multicultural education* (sometimes referred to as cultural pluralist) phase. These phases were often overlapping.

4.1.1 Assimilation

At the heart of this phase (from the 1960s to the early 1970s) was the idea that absorption into the dominant or 'host' society/culture should be the primary target. As one official report put it:

> half a million immigrants represent a small proportion of the total population of Britain. But these immigrants are visibly distinguishable by the colour of their skins, and many come from societies whose habits and customs are very different from those in Britain. …
>
> … a national system of education must aim at producing citizens who can take their place in society properly equipped to exercise rights and perform duties which are the same as those of other citizens. If their parents were brought up in another culture or another tradition, children should be encouraged to respect it, but a national system cannot be expected to perpetuate the different values of immigrant groups.
>
> (Commonwealth Immigrants Advisory Council, 1964, pp.624–5)

Later, a circular from the Department of Education and Science (DES) (1965) said: 'it is inevitable that, as the proportion of immigrant children in a school or class increases the problems will become more difficult to solve and the chances of assimilation more remote'. Underlying such statements is the idea that the British nation is, or was, a single homogeneous entity, having a common heritage which gave rise to cultural indivisibility. Assimilation in this context was deemed to be the most appropriate means of guaranteeing cultural and social stability in the face of 'alien' presences.

What policy instruments, then, could be introduced to deal with the 'problem' and ensure speedy and orderly assimilation? Three such instruments were devised:

1   A system of collecting statistics, introduced in 1966. Information was gathered on children who had migrated to this country themselves or who had been

born in the UK to parents who had migrated to the UK in the previous 10 years. These statistics then underpinned:

2   A system of disbursing funds known as Section 11 money, from central government to those local authorities in England and Wales which had what was termed a 'substantial number' of Commonwealth immigrants within their boundaries; and:

3   A system of dispersal of black pupils around borough schools as a means of preventing their over-concentration. This system of dispersal became known popularly as 'bussing' after a similar system instituted in the USA, a country which was believed to have much to teach the UK now that it had what was regarded as a large black presence.

The example of bussing

In 1963 the Commonwealth Immigrants Advisory Council (CIAC) recommended to the Home Office that school catchment areas should, 'where necessary', be adjusted to ensure a 'racial' balance. Where such adjustment was not sufficient to ensure the appropriate degree of dispersal of 'immigrant' children then bussing should be implemented. Meanwhile, some white parents in the outer west London town of Southall, in the Borough of Ealing, began to complain to the local education authority (LEA) about 'swamping' of local primary schools by 'immigrant' children (Campaign Against Racism and Fascism/Southall Rights, 1981). Their agitation resulted in the LEA sending a delegation to the then Conservative Minister of Education Sir Edward Boyle, who in October 1963 visited Southall in an attempt to reassure and calm the local white population. The incoming Labour government of 1964 reaffirmed the commitment to a policy of dispersal in its (in)famous Circular 7/65 (entitled *The Education of Immigrants*, Department of Education and Science, 1965).

This document enshrined the upper limit of 33 per cent 'immigrant' pupil presence in any one school in official DES policy. However, because the main onus of responsibility for the arrangements and provision of schooling fell on local education authorities, DES policy did not always translate into LEA practice. The Inner London Education Authority (ILEA) and Birmingham LEA, for example, were two authorities with 'substantial numbers of immigrants' which had decided against the implementation of central government policy on dispersal, opting instead for alternative measures. Yet Townsend (1971), in research on LEA responses to the presence of black pupils, found that 11 out of the 33 authorities surveyed, including Ealing, Bradford and Blackburn, were in fact operating a policy of dispersal.

In Ealing, the local authority responsible for Southall, 15 per cent of the school-age population were classed as immigrant in 1964. The vast majority of these were of south Asian origin or descent, with only 100 out of a total of 1,130 being of West Indian origin or descent. The Campaign Against Racism and Fascism (CARF) and Southall Rights found that, even in the 1970s, the figures for bussing were as follows:

■   1973: 100 mainly Asian children;

■   1976: 2,500 mainly Asian children, with an additional 400 making their own way to schools other than their local one;

■ 1979: 1,500 children still being dispersed despite official abandonment of the policy.

The implementation of a dispersal policy in Southall/Ealing can be seen to result from the convergence of views between central government, local government and some, particularly vociferous, white parents. Black parents, however, were less than happy, raising the question about which parents had a voice in the development and implementation of policy. By the late 1960s many of those whose children were being bussed all around the borough refused to co-operate and in 1969 the Indian Workers Association organized a sustained campaign against the practice: 'The campaign emphasized not only the disadvantages the bussed children suffered and the poor education they received, but also the ways in which the segregation of the children created and perpetuated the hostility and racialism which led to attacks on them, both verbal and physical' (Campaign Against Racism and Fascism/Southall Rights, 1981, p.33).

ACTIVITY 3.5

Extract 3.3 comes from the speech made to the House of Commons by Sir Edward Boyle (then Minister of Education) in the heat of the controversy about 'bussing' and after his visit to Southall. Read through this extract carefully and, as you do so, think about what evidence is given for the following ideas:

1   That black pupils were viewed as a problem.

2   That 30 per cent represents the educationally tolerable upper limit for the presence of black pupils in any one school.

3   That inequality is a natural rather than a social phenomenon.

Does the speech suggest that the problem posed by the presence of black pupils will be short-lived? If not, what does this imply about the 'problem' being posed as one of the newly arrived status of some of the black pupils?

Extract 3.3 Boyle: 'Speech to House of Commons, 1963'

I think that perhaps especially in the week of President Kennedy's death I must at the start state to the House my own belief that the problem of racial relations, and of integration versus segregation, will continue for generations to be one of the most important facing the free world. …

The school is, therefore, of great importance as the obvious instrument for achieving integration.

I am not, of course, directly responsible for running the schools, but my approach to this is a very simple one. It seems to me that I am responsible quite clearly to this House for all children who are resident in this country, whatever their intelligence, whatever their race or colour, and receiving education according to their age and ability. …

… [W]hen we advocate educational advance … we say very truly today that our children tend to be more equal as physical specimens than they ever were before … but the opportunities children have in their homes for learning and gaining knowledge of England can be very unequal; and just as they can be unequal as between native children, as one says so often, so there are greater inequalities of opportunity between native children and immigrant children. …

So far as I can influence these matters at all it is my own hope that schools will not become segregated. ... I am sure that that is wrong for two reasons.

In the first place, in the interests of the general policy for racial integration, it is my view that efforts must be made to prevent individual schools from becoming only immigrant schools. Secondly, there is the educational point of which we must not lose sight. If possible, it is desirable on educational grounds that no one school should have more than about 30 per cent. of immigrants. ... I am sure that the educational problems that one gets above the level of 30 per cent. immigrant children become infinitely harder and perhaps impossible to tackle.

Let us be under no illusions as to how difficult the problem is from the point of view of local education authorities ... For example, one must realise the difficulty in places where nearly a whole neighbourhood is taken over by immigrant families. The school serving the neighbourhood will cease to have a sufficient supply of native children, and it is both politically and legally more or less impossible to compel native parents to send their children to a school in an immigrant area if there are places for them in other schools. Moreover, even when native parents continue to live alongside immigrants, they will often seek to transfer their children to more distant non-immigrant schools if their local school has more than about 30 per cent. of immigrant children. ...

One must recognise the perfectly legitimate anxiety of many of the parents of what I call the native children; one must recognise the reasonable fear of many parents that their children will get less than a fair share of the teachers' attention when a great deal of it must of necessity be given both to language teaching and to the social training of immigrant children.

So I say, on the general principle, by all means let us stand firmly in this House against segregation between native school and immigrant schools. ... But let us realise at the same time the legitimate fears of parents of native-born children and let us very fully realise the particular problems, administrative problems not least, with which any local authority will be faced. ...

My Department is due to meet the Middlesex and Southall education authorities in December to work out arrangements for distributing Indian and Pakistani children over the schools of the borough. I must regretfully tell the House that one school ... must be regarded now as irretrievably an immigrant school. The important thing to do is to prevent this happening elsewhere. ...

I want to make one or two remarks about the practical steps that can be taken. I take account of the need for extra teachers to cope with immigrants by giving the authorities concerned additions to their teacher quotas. ...

I certainly will support any authority which tries to spread immigrant children by introducing zoning schemes. This must be a matter of co-operation rather than compulsion, but I can promise any authority which attempts to spread immigrant children my strongest support ...

Let us remember that the present immigrant settlers will produce an increasing number of children. Immigrant children as they reach maturity may well reproduce in larger numbers than perhaps some other parts of the population. This is not just a short-term matter, but a long-term question as well. It affects secondary as well as primary education.

(*Hansard*, 25 November–6 December 1963, cols 438–44)

COMMENT

The starting-point for seeing black pupils being constructed as a problem is the very fact that there was such a speech made in the House of Commons. Also indicative is the tone of the speech, which suggests a state of great urgency, and the idea that the 'problem of race relations' will continue for a long time, which together suggest that the UK now faces a 'problem' which must be brought under 'control' without further delay. There is also the fact that a need for 'dispersal' or 'bussing' of black pupils was deemed necessary at all. This immediately casts these children as 'different' – and it is a 'difference' which needs to be kept under strict management. Indeed, this idea is carried even more starkly by the suggestion that a great catastrophe would befall a school were it to become an 'immigrant' school.

Yet no evidence is given to suggest the 'educational' reasons for limiting the numbers to no more than 30 per cent. Instead, this limit seems to be necessary to appease 'native' (an interesting reverse of colonial discourse) parents, who have a 'reasonable fear', and local education authorities who will have to 'manage' the problem.

In part this 'problem' to be 'managed' arises because of the inequalities of opportunity to which it gives rise. But there is no suggestion as to the cause of such inequality of opportunity and so it is implied that it is a 'natural' or essential result of racial difference, rather than a socially produced inequality about which schools (and other public institutions) can do something.

Moreover, it appears from this speech that it is a 'problem' that will have to be managed for a long time to come. This we can see from the reference at the end of the extract about the assumed population growth of the 'immigrant' populations. This, then, undermines the idea that it is just newly arrived status, or ability in the English language, that is the issue. Behind this, therefore, is a suggestion that the 'difference' between 'native' and 'immigrant' is one which is persistent and fixed – again it is constructed as essential.

From this it can be seen that these ideas about the presence of black pupils in British schools are mapped on to a rather contradictory construction of British society. On the one hand, it is clear that there is some recognition of the inequalities which exist among 'native' (meaning white) children. However, this inequality is not a matter of the systemic social divisions which accompany class divisions because the inequalities reside in the home. On the other hand, the UK, if understood as a white society (its 'natives') is also constructed as homogeneous – a homogeneity which could be undermined in the presence of 'immigrant' populations – hence the need to restrict the numbers of pupils in any one school from these populations.

Extract 3.3 is particularly helpful for:

■ Demonstrating the tenor of the assimilationist phase of education policy, and the essentialisms which racial classifications carry.   essentialism

■ Showing how 'the nation' was constructed as homogeneous and white and that the task was to ensure that this homogeneity was not disrupted by the presence of pupils constructed as racially 'Other'.

■ Providing an illustration of the links between the social construction of racial groups and boundaries and the ways in which public debates and policies both reflect and rework particular conceptions of social problems.

■ ■ ■

We now move on to look at what has been termed the 'integrationist' phase of education policy in order to explore these themes further.

4.1.2   Integration

As the 1960s passed into the 1970s many involved in the world of compulsory education, as policy makers, teachers or government inspectors, began to challenge the assimilationist model on many different grounds. These ranged from the opposition by black parents to 'bussing' through to the idea that, whilst the objectives of assimilation were laudable and necessary, the methods were ineffective and intolerant of the cultural diversity which black settlement had brought. This idea of the importance of tolerance of diversity was summed up in a phrase of the then Labour Home Secretary Roy Jenkins (1966), when he said that what was needed was 'not a flattening process of assimilation but equal opportunity, accompanied by cultural diversity, in an atmosphere of mutual tolerance'.

However, this call to tolerance of diversity was not the same thing as an abandonment of the overall goals of the assimilation project, as one education inspector made clear:

> Contrary to the assimilationist belief that, given English language fluency, the immigrant would disappear into the crowd, those arguing for integration claimed that a much more planned and detailed education and social programme needed to be undertaken if immigrants were to be able to integrate with the majority society. The emphasis was still upon integrating the minorities with the majority society and culture so that a culturally homogeneous society would be created. This meant that it was up to the minorities to change and adapt, and there was little or no pressure upon the majority society to modify or change its prevailing attitudes or practices. However, to enable integration to take place, it was argued that the majority society needed to be more aware of historical and cultural factors affecting different minorities. Knowledge and awareness would enable the majority society to make allowances for differences in lifestyle, culture and religion that might make it difficult for some immigrant groups to integrate with British society and would help to avoid the embarrassing mistakes that could arise from ignorance.
>
> (Bolton, 1979, pp.4–5)

The aims of integration were the same as those of assimilation. Both approaches were premised on the belief that, with the exception of the areas of black settlement, the UK was a homogeneous society; that black children and their parents must be absorbed into that homogeneous society; and that this must be done with as little disruption to the 'host' society as possible. What had changed was the idea about *how* these objectives could be achieved. The starting-point was that understanding and knowledge about these 'other' cultures was required and those most in need of this understanding were teachers themselves. As a result, a characteristic feature of the 'integrationist' phase was the proliferation of in-service courses in cultural awareness – a practice which often involved visits by top ranking or specialist teachers to the Caribbean and the Indian sub-continent in pursuit of cultural understanding and sensitization. Begun in education, this model was soon to proliferate to other welfare services, including the police and social services. R. Street-Porter points out that, whilst the statement made by Roy Jenkins about integration recognizes the problems of the assimilationist model and the need to accept cultural diversity, the model of:

Cultural integration seems to have been accepted merely as a modest tokenism, an acceptance of that which is quaint in a minority culture but a worried rejection of those cultural aspects that seem not just alien but threateningly so. In other words, minority groups in practice are allowed complete freedom to define their own cultural identity only in so far as this does not conflict with that of the white indigenous community. …

This gap between the idealism expressed by Roy Jenkins and the practical implementation of integrationist policies is clearly shown in educational practice. The late sixties saw the start of several small policies which reflected partly the views of the Jenkins statement and also the assimilationist hangover. Teachers saw the need to become more informed about the cultural background of the minority group children they taught, but the motivation to do this was still to assist in easing the children into the unchanging culture of the school. There was a mushrooming of courses and conferences to inform teachers about the homelands of such *British-born* children and there was an increasing number of advisory posts created to deal with the 'problems' of 'immigrant' education.

(The Open University, 1978, pp.80–1, emphasis added)

At its core, then, the integrationist model still had a commitment to promoting social and cultural stability in a framework in which 'black' is equated with 'problem', 'British' is equated with 'white' and 'Britain'/'the UK' is equated with homogeneity.

Why do you think we added emphasis to the term 'British-born' in the quotation above?

The reference to 'British-born children' emphasizes the way in which the integrationist model continued to exclude black pupils from its notions of 'the British' or 'the nation'. Place of birth and the overall social and cultural environment in which black children, as well as white, live their lives is only secondary in this approach because colour and the national origins of their parents are seen as the primary determinant of these children's value systems, behaviours and beliefs.

4.1.3   Multicultural and anti-racist education

By the 1980s the intersection of education policy and practice and racializing discourse was taking place on different terrain from that which had provided the context for either the assimilationist (expressed in its most pronounced form in the practice of 'bussing') or integrationist models. Before going on to consider the dominant ways in which 'race' was constructed in the multicultural and anti-racist approaches to education policy we should take a moment to consider an important point.

By the 1980s it had become apparent that the black presence in the UK was now a permanent one as most people, black and white, now realized. One effect of this realization was a change in the word most commonly applied to black people in both official and popular discourse. By the 1980s it was much more common to hear black individuals and groups referred to as 'ethnic minorities' rather than as 'immigrants'. This is not to say that the word 'immigrant' fell out of use altogether, but it became more common to use the term 'ethnic minority' or even 'the ethnic communities'. For social scientists working within a social constructionist framework this change in name is important because it suggests that a different kind or type of social 'subject' has been constructed.

An 'immigrant' is a subject who is viewed as a foreigner who has come into a pre-existing community – a nation. This is not just a legal position (as we saw earlier): it is also a social one. The boundary of social difference and exclusion is constructed from a distinct set of criteria related to the political and geographical borders which demarcate 'the people' of the nation-state. An 'ethnic minority' is quite another 'subject'. She or he is already defined as 'inside' the political and geographical borders of the nation-state, perhaps with full legal citizenship. The boundary of social difference in the case of the 'ethnic minority' tends, then, to be constituted out of racial or cultural features which are distinct from those that are said to characterize the majority or 'the people'. An 'ethnic minority' is 'in' the nation (and may well have been for generations), but not 'of' the nation in the way that this is understood as an 'imagined community'. In addition, Mercer (1993, p.295) has noted that the 'ethnic minority' is also a minor in the sense that a child is constructed as minor: that is, without a voice, in need of protection and in need of control.

Three important points can be derived from this change in naming:

1   It reflects a change in the type of racialized subject that is constructed.

2   Accompanying this change is a shift in the terms on which their difference or 'Otherness' is constructed. This 'racialized subject' is no longer the 'immigrant' who must learn to do in Rome as the Romans do, but rather a category of person who, or group which, has distinct abilities and needs which must be met, but which are subordinate to those of the 'majority'.

3   The 'majority' is constructed as the norm, but a norm without ethnicity.

This shift is important because it provides the context in which the debate about multicultural education (MCE) and anti-racist education (ARE) occurred. This reconstitution of racialized groups did not mean that 'race' was no longer considered to be an educational issue. Rather, the terms of the debate had been shifted by the efforts of those within education and the black populations to place multicultural and/or anti-racist education on the agenda.

Although what is meant by the term 'multicultural education' has been the subject of a long and often strident debate, it is possible to identify two main strands common to its various versions: first, that education policy and practice must attend to the needs of 'ethnic minority' children; and second, that a multicultural UK requires that *all* children are prepared for life in such a society. That these efforts met with some success is evidenced by both the number of LEAs which adopted some form of multicultural, anti-racist, or equal opportunities policies; and, at central government level, the publication by the then Department of Education and Science of the report entitled *Education for All* (the Swann Report) in 1985. This legitimated MCE as the most appropriate form for compulsory education in England and Wales. As a result, to some limited extent the issue of 'race' and education became recast as that of 'racism within education', and gave some legitimacy to the idea that the conception and delivery of education reproduced the racist marginalization of those cast as 'racially' or 'culturally' Other. This was a considerable move away from the two former approaches which had had the effect of continuing to cast black pupils as outside of, or excluded from, the 'British nation or people'. Thus 'in challenging the structural and cultural marginalization of Britain's black minority communities, they also began to shift the terms around which British national identities had

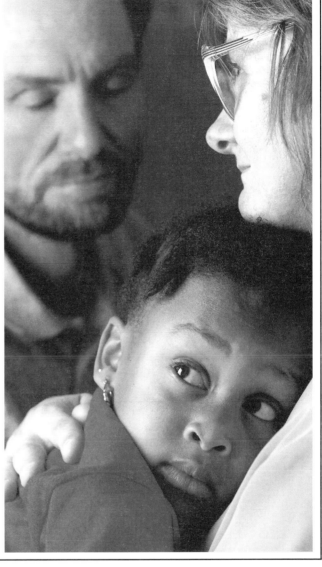

Kamal Ahmed on a dispute over fostering

British life 'may harm' girl, 4

A FOUR-YEAR-OLD black child who has lived her whole life in Britain faces deportation to Jamaica with her mother this week after a court ruling said she would be disadvantaged by being brought up by a white foster family.

(*The Guardian*, 14 October 1996, p.6)

What makes a Briton?
Colour, place of birth or ancestry?

sedimented over the years of colonial domination and imperial grandeur' (Rattansi, 1992, p.11).

But if this was the result of the shift to a multicultural approach to education in the 1980s it did not mean that education policy and practice in relation to 'race' and ethnicity were devoid of contentious debate. This debate and disagreement took place around a distinction which was made between multicultural education and anti-racist education and is related to which of the two terms was to be used as the focus of policy development and practice. This mattered because the name given affected what was opened up to, or closed off from, debate. We can begin to make sense of this by looking at a concrete example.

In 1979 a government Committee of Inquiry was established under the chairmanship of Lord Rampton to look into the 'Causes of underachievement of children of West Indian origin'. This Committee published an interim report (the Rampton Report) in 1981 entitled *West Indian Children in Our Schools.* The Committee continued its investigations under Lord Swann from that time and delivered its final report (*Education for All*, known as the Swann Report) in 1985. Both parts of the Committee's investigations took place under the following terms of reference:

> Recognising the contribution of schools in preparing all pupils for life in a society which is both multi-racial and culturally diverse, the Committee is required to:
>
> > review in relation to schools the educational needs and attainments of children from ethnic minority groups taking account, as necessary, of factors outside the formal education system relevant to school performance, including influences in early childhood and prospects for school leavers;
> >
> > consider the potential value of instituting arrangements for keeping under review the educational performance of different ethnic minority groups, and what those arrangements might be …
>
> > (Department of Education and Science, 1985, p.vii)

ACTIVITY 3.6

Extracts 3.4 and 3.5 are taken from the evidence given to the Committee of Inquiry by the Institute of Race Relations (IRR) and The Swann Report respectively. Read these extracts now and list the points of contrast and comparison between them. Pay particular attention to the relative emphases given to issues of 'race', racism and culture in each. How appropriate do you think the argument between them is for school education in the UK today?

Extract 3.4 Institute of Race Relations: 'IRR statement to the Rampton Committee on Education'

1 In making our submission to your Committee we must confess our inability to speak directly to your terms of reference, because of the way the problem has been posed. …

2 Your terms of reference are concerned with 'the educational needs and attainments of children from all ethnic minority groups', particularly West Indian children. We feel, however, that an ethnic or cultural approach to the educational needs and attainments of racial minorities evades the fundamental reasons for their disabilities – which are the racialist attitudes and the racist practices in the larger society and in the educational system itself.

3 Ethnic minorities, we would submit, do not suffer disabilities because of ethnic differences as such (if they did, we would be addressing ourselves to the ethnic differences of white society as well) but because such differences are given differential weightage in a system of racial hierarchy.

4 That is not to say that the differences in language, customs, values, etc. of different ethnic groups cannot be mediated by the educational system and even help to change attitudes, but to say that such mediation is content to tinker with educational techniques and methods and leaves unaltered the racist fabric of the educational system. And education itself comes to be seen in terms of an adjustment process within a racialist society and not as a force for changing the values that make that society racialist.

5   Our concern therefore is not centrally with multicultural, multiethnic education, but with anti-racist education (which by its very nature would include the study of other cultures). Just to learn about other peoples' cultures, though, is not to learn about the racism of one's own. To learn about the racism of one's own culture, on the other hand, is to approach other cultures objectively. …

8   [Development of new anti-racist teaching materials] would have to reach the core of racist beliefs, would have to show, for example, that civilisations rise and fall and none is 'superior' for all time; that racialism, like most cultural phenomena, is the concomitant of a particular economic system, which received its main and most sustained impetus in the historical period of colonialism.

This Institute … [will] produce … materials which will radically re-examine white society and history in the light of the black experience.

In thus dealing seriously with an alternative view of the nature and development of British society these materials we hope would help pupils, both black and white … to develop a critical judgement, not only of their own beliefs and values, but of contemporary social institutions, prevailing attitudes, orthodoxies past and present, and their inter-relationship with the actual structure of society.

(Institute of Race Relations, 1980, pp.81–3)

Extract 3.5 Department of Education and Science: 'Education for all'

We believe it is essential to change fundamentally the terms of the debate about the educational response to today's multi-racial society and to look ahead to educating *all* children, from whatever ethnic group, to an understanding of the shared values of our society as a whole as well as to an appreciation of the diversity of lifestyles and cultural, religious and linguistic backgrounds which make up this society and the wider world. In so doing, all pupils should be given the knowledge and skills needed not only to contribute positively to shaping the future nature of British society but also to determine their own individual identities, free from preconceived or imposed stereotypes of their 'place' in that society. We believe that schools also however have a responsibility, within the tradition of a flexible and child-orientated education system, to meet individual educational needs of *all* pupils in a positive and supportive manner, and this would include catering for any particular educational needs which an ethnic minority pupil may have, arising for example from his or her linguistic or cultural background. …

'Education for All' describes … the approach to education which we wish to put forward, since it reflects the responsibility which we feel that all those concerned with education share in laying the foundations for the kind of pluralist society which we envisaged …

A 'Good' Education

[A 'good' education is established on the premise that:]

Education for diversity and for social and racial harmony suggests that the richness of cultural variety in Britain … should be appreciated and utilised in education curricula at all levels. This can only have beneficial effects for all students in widening cultural awareness and in developing sensitivity towards the cultural identity and practices of various groups.

[CNAA Multicultural Working Group]

We also see education as having a major role to play in countering the racism which still persists in Britain today and which we believe constitutes one of the chief obstacles to the realisation of a truly pluralist society. ...

[Thus] [t]he role of education cannot be and cannot be expected to be to reinforce the values, beliefs and cultural identity which each child brings to school ... We would instead wish to see schools encouraging the cultural *development* of all their pupils, both in terms of helping them to gain confidence in their own cultural identities while learning to respect the identities of other groups as equally valid in their own right.

(Department of Education and Science, 1985, pp.316–23)

COMMENT

In our 'reading' of these extracts we can begin by identifing the main arguments of each. In the statement from the IRR the following points seemed to be most explicit:

1   It puts at the fore the issue of *racism* and the *inequalities* to which it gives rise.

2   These racist inequalities are said to *reside* in both education and the wider society.

3   In this context 'difference' is of social and educational significance because it is *hierarchically* ordered.

4   Such ordering is *racial* ordering – that is, it is to do with the marking of *bodies* because of, for example, skin colour; it is not to do with culture.

5   Attending to cultural differences does not get to the *structural* factors which produce racism.

6   As such, educational practice should focus on racism and the *forces* which produce and sustain it.

7   This would include pointing out that national or imperial power is a *historically specific formation* – as opposed to a consequence of genetic endowment of the people of a nation – and as such will always be subject to challenge and change.

8   Racism is itself cultural and is a reflection of an *economic system*.

9   Racism as culture structures or *fashions the curriculum*, which, in its turn, reproduces racism.

10 The focus of examination should be *white society* from the *standpoint of black experience*.

Underlying this last statement is a particular view about the nature of British society in the 1980s and this view can be characterized as containing the following elements:

■   British society is fundamentally unequal in that it is organized around relations of subordination and domination and as such racism is systemic.

■   The systemic root of all these relations, including those organized around a racial hierarchy, is an economic system.

■   Change therefore must be systemic.

In sharp contrast to the IRR statement, the Swann Report begins from a very different position. One 'reading' of it seems to suggest the following main points:

1   Rather than emphasizing 'race' or 'racism' it focuses on *ethnic diversity* in contemporary England and Wales.

2   Given this, no pupils' *identity* or *place* in society should develop according to *stereotypes*.

3   This means that education must meet the needs of *all* pupils, and, where necessary, take account of any *ethnically derived* needs.

4   The term 'education for all' reflects this focus.

5   Cultural diversity is *enriching* and should be *valued* and *used* as a *curriculum resource*.

6   It is in this context that *racism* must be *challenged* because it prevents such value being given to cultural diversity.

7   Whilst cultural diversity must be valued, *no one* culture must be given a special or *privileged* place in the school environment or curriculum.

As with the IRR statement there is an underlying assumption within the Swann Report about the nature of British society, which can be summed up in the following points:

- The UK today is a pluralist society, which means that it is made up of a mix of social groups which can be demarcated according to specific characteristics – in this case cultural characteristics.

- It is also a meritocratic society at root, which means that ability and effort are rewarded.

- Therefore the idea that British society is fundamentally organized through structured inequality is missing from this perspective.

- Consequently, racism is not a systemic or organic part of British society, but is, rather, an 'accidental' feature of it which must be attended to.

It is possible to derive much of this perspective from the extract from the Swann Report with which we have been working. However, unlike the IRR statement which is a short document, the Swann Report has an added advantage in that we can go to other parts of it to look for further evidence as to the interpretation of its underlying perspective. One such example is in the Report's discussion of 'institutional racism':

> We see institutional racism as describing the way in which a range of long established systems, practices and procedures, both within education and the wider society, which were originally conceived and devised to meet the needs and aspirations of a relatively homogeneous society, can now be seen not only to fail to take account of the multi-racial nature of Britain today but may also ignore or even actively work against the interests of ethnic minority communities.
>
> (Department of Education and Science, 1985, p.28)

This clearly shows the assumption of a meritocracy and the absence of any systemic and intentional racism. It also shows that the approach centres on the need for change which has emerged as a result of the heterogeneity which now characterizes the UK, and which was assumed to be absent before. It suggests that this heterogeneity is only understood in terms of ethnic diversity (though it is notable that in this passage the term 'multi-racial' is used), which emerged with the post-1945 black presence, and therefore, previous to this time, constructs a UK devoid of other major cleavages such as those deriving from class or gender.

■ ■ ■

Summary

The statements illustrated in Extracts 3.4 and 3.5 were characteristic of a divergence in perspective about the relationship between education policy and practice on the one hand, and 'race', ethnicity and racism on the other, which were known as the 'anti-racist or multicultural education' debates. As with all such debates about the development of policy and its deployment into practice, this debate was far ranging, complex and highly contentious. The main points which distinguish the two approaches are addressed in the two extracts.

Two further issues addressed by the debate are of relevance here. First, oppositional strategies and discourses which were intended to contest the racial and/or ethnic subordinations, which are themselves produced by the prevailing social, cultural, economic and political relations, can also lead to racial or ethnic exclusions. We will consider this by looking a little further at the 'anti-racist' perspective. Second, exclusions can result from the application of prescriptive policy formulations aimed at addressing racial inequality. We will consider this by examining some aspects of a document called the Burnage Report.

5 The 'anti-racist' perspective and its exclusions

We have seen that at the centre of the 'anti-racist' perspective was the issue of racism. Added to this, however, was a notion of something called 'the black experience', the defining feature of which was seen to be racism. In earlier sections we have looked at some of the ways in which racism serves to limit access to welfare services and benefits for many black people, but to suggest that racism is the defining feature of black experience raises a number of other points which it is important to consider. First, it suggests that there is only one black experience, undifferentiated along lines of gender, class, sexuality or, indeed, ethnic distinction *within* black communities. In other words it constructs a homogeneous black community and closes off recognition of (and challenge to) relations of subordination and domination 'internal' to these communities.

These closures or exclusions arose out of a discourse of 'blackness' since this sought to deny the well-established negative associations which the idea of 'blackness' carried. The discourse of 'blackness' also sought to disrupt a long established feature of British imperial rule: the divide-and-rule tactics which served to construct hard boundaries and divisions between the African, the Caribbean and the Asian. In terms of this oppositional discourse, 'black' signalled a common social position and experience in contemporary Britain, the roots of which lay in the colonial past. 'Black' in this sense was understood as a *political* colour rather than one connected to any particular body type. In other words, being 'black' was not based on physical variation among human bodies, but on a historical and contemporary location in a system of global and national relations. Those who could claim a place within this discourse were all those of Asian, African and Caribbean origin or descent, and, for some activists, also those of Arab and Latin American origin or descent. It was, then, an attempt at constructing a discourse and practice of opposition around an inclusive category.

Rattansi (1992) has pointed out that 'black' in this incarnation was a category of *representation* which sought to emphasize particular experiences around which 'Afro–Asian' unity could be constructed, and has examined the exclusions which can emerge when a collectivity is imagined in this way. In this idea of 'black' there is no room for members of those ethnic groups assumed to belong to 'black' to have a varying range of experiences – they are reduced to a single category. The logical consequence is that those who have different experiences, or understand their location in British society in different ways, become excluded from view.

Exclusion also arises from the ways in which colour is used to construct boundaries of belonging. For while 'black' was to be disconnected from its association with people of African and African-Caribbean origin or descent, skin colour retained a privileged position. Thus 'non-white' skin remained the feature around which racism was experienced and this had the effect of excluding other groups of people, such as Jewish people, who could make a claim on 'whiteness' but who nevertheless were just as racialized as the various black populations.

The 'anti-racist education' perspective therefore led to its own exclusions organized around the representational categories at its heart. The paradoxical effect of this was that 'the black community' was constructed as homogeneous and so the 'anti-racist' perspective excluded from its view those black people whose experiences were structured by more than just racism – by gender or sexuality, for example. Similarly, it excluded white groups whose experiences were also structured by processes of racialization, a point to which we shall return in section 7.

5.1   The Burnage Report

The Burnage Report (1989), entitled *Murder in the Playground*, provides an illustration of the issues raised in this latter debate. What is significant about this Report is that it was written by a group of panellists who had distinguished records in the struggle to challenge racism within education and yet it heavily criticized the operation of anti-racist policies within the school. For our purposes what is relevant is the Report's concern about the ways in which a *particular version* of anti-racism had the effect of repositioning people in racialized discourses and social relations which resulted in racial marginalizations. It also gives a clear example of the ways in which *white people*, as well as black, are positioned by racializing discourse. It is these points that are highlighted in what follows. Before you read on, it is worth pointing out that you may find some of the detail of the events described alarming and upsetting. You should, however, persevere as the incidents that the inquiry was set up to investigate make it very clear that social constructions, and the policies they underwrite, have 'real' effects on everyday life. Remember that the key points to look for are:

1   How boundaries of 'race' were constructed in this case.

2   For which groups racism was considered to be an issue.

3   The exclusions that resulted.

The Burnage Report is a 530-page document detailing the process, evidence and conclusions of a Panel of Inquiry into racism and racial violence in

Manchester schools. The circumstances leading to the inquiry were the death of Ahmed Iqbal Ullah at Burnage High School in September 1986 after he had been knifed by a fellow school pupil named Darren Coulburn.

5.1.1 The incident and its surrounding circumstances

The following points concerning the circumstances of Ahmed Iqbal Ullah's death are adapted from Chapter 2 of the Burnage Report:

1   15 September 1986 and the new school year begins. Four Asian boys are playing football at break-time when Darren Coulburn takes the ball and throws it on a roof. The four boys threaten to tell the deputy head teacher and he gives the ball back. As he does so he threatens one of the boys with a beating up after school.

2   At the end of the day Darren Coulburn waits for the boy he had threatened earlier and punches and kicks him and subjects the boy to taunts which carry with them the history of racial subservience by making the boy stand and sit and say 'sorry master'.

3   Ahmed Ullah sees this and intervenes, a thing he often did. Ahmed Ullah now makes Darren Coulburn perform the humiliating act of standing and sitting, thus reversing the order of dominance.

4   16 September and rumour spreads throughout the school that there is to be a fight between Darren Coulburn and Ahmed Ullah at the end of the day. This begins with much crowd encouragement from other boys in the school. Ahmed Ullah bleeds from injuries he sustains but generally 'wins' the fight. Darren Coulburn runs off chased by Ahmed Ullah, but older boys and then teachers intervene and the fight and chase end.

5   Ahmed Ullah goes home feeling 'victorious' despite his cuts and bruises and tells his mother that Darren Coulburn had threatened to kill him. This alarms his mother but he shrugs it off. Meanwhile on the same evening Darren Coulburn is asked by a friend about the fight and he says it was 'just a fight' but adds 'let him start again and I'll stab him' (p.14).

6   Wednesday 17 September and Ahmed Ullah's mother does not want Ahmed to go to school until she has had a chance to talk to the teacher. Ahmed Ullah tells her not to worry and eventually she lets him go to school, feeling reassured that trouble among the boys from the school only starts after school and not before it and by the end of the day she will have spoken to the teacher.

7   Meanwhile Darren Coulburn is also going to school and after telling more boys about the fight the previous evening, he shows them a knife and repeats his threat to stab Ahmed Ullah if another fight starts.

8   The two boys meet up in the school and a group of boys begin to urge them to fight. Darren Coulburn appears to want to avoid the fight but Ahmed Ullah seems keen to have it and pushes Darren Coulburn. 'Darren then turned and bent over – the next instant he stabbed Ahmed in the stomach, the blade came out covered in blood. Ahmed staggered away and fell. As he did so one eye-witness heard Darren Coulburn shout "Do you want

another one, you stupid Paki; there's plenty more where that came from".
Another remembers "You want it again, Paki?" before Darren ran off. A few
minutes later he was seen by fourth and fifth year students at the gates of
the upper school freaking out, running about and saying "I've killed a Paki".
Ahmed lay in the playground. Darren had run off. It was approximately
8.30 a.m.' (p.15).

9   On arrival at hospital at 9.10 a.m. Ahmed Ullah was pronounced clinically
    dead and was not able to be resuscitated.

This was an extreme and tragic event, but Table 3.1, taken from a 1996 Office
for Standards in Education (OFSTED) Report, indicates that racial violence within
schools is far from an isolated occurrence.

Table 3.1   A brief chronology of racial violence against children and young people

1991

February: Rolan Adams, a 15-year-old black grammar school pupil from south London, is stabbed to
            death by a young neo-Nazi on the Thamesmead estate

1992

July: Rohit Duggal, a 16-year-old Asian pupil, is stabbed to death during a confrontation with a
            group of white youths in Greenwich, south London

October: Gangs of white and Asian youths involved in violent clashes outside Shawlands Academy,
            Glasgow

1993

April: Black sixth-former Stephen Lawrence, 18, is stabbed to death by half a dozen white youths

April: 14-year-old black Sheffield boy bayonets Grant Jackson, a 17-year-old white boy, to death
            during inter-school gang warfare

May: Two Bengali youths, aged 17, are attacked with a machete by a skinhead as they sit on a wall
            outside one of their homes in Camden, north London

September: Quaddus Ali, a 17-year-old Bangladeshi student at Tower Hamlets College, east London, is
            savagely beaten by a group of white men, including skinheads

September: At least nine pupils transfer from George Green's School on the Isle of Dogs, Tower Hamlets,
            because of racial harassment

1994

February: Muktar Ahmed, 19, savagely beaten by a gang of 20 white youths in Bethnal Green, east
            London. A few days later, a group of white youths armed with iron bars and accompanied by
            dogs attack Asian students sitting in a park during their lunch break from Tower Hamlets
            College. The following day a 14-year-old Bengali boy is stabbed in the face by four white
            men as he walks down Bethnal Green Road

March: Violent clashes take place between black and Asian youths, some of them armed, in and
            around Quintin Kynaston School in St John's Wood, north London

June: Student Shah Mohammed Ruhul Alam, 17, is critically wounded after being stabbed by 10
            white youths

August: Richard Everitt, a 15-year-old white pupil, is stabbed to death by a group of 11 Asian youths
            near King's Cross Station, north London

December: The National Union of Students launches a 24-hour hotline to tackle growing harassment and
            intimidation of students by far-Right groups

Source: based on OFSTED, 1996, p.51

Here we will focus on (i) the ways in which the members of the Panel of Inquiry, all associated with an 'anti-racist' perspective, criticized the particular model of 'anti-racism' and a *particular style* of implementation instituted at Burnage High School (Gordon and Rosenberg, 1989, p.47); and (ii) the exclusions which resulted from this model and style.

The starting-point for the criticisms made by the Report's authors (the panellists) was their understanding of the concept of racism. Racism, they suggested, is:

> the doctrine that an individual or his or her behaviour is determined by stable, inherited characteristics deriving from separate racial stocks, having distinctive attributes, and usually standing in relations of 'superiority' and 'inferiority' ... When these [ideas] become systematized into a philosophy of 'race' superiority, and when this then becomes a part of the way in which society as a whole is organized, then the term 'racism' is used.
>
> (The Burnage Report, 1989, p.43)

An individual can be called racist if he or she subscribes to such a doctrine, and equally her or his behaviour can be defined as racist if it is based on such a doctrine '*or if it reflects the racist nature of society*' (p.44). From this definition the panellists were then able to designate the murder of Ahmed Ullah as racist, *not* because of the *motive*, but rather because of 'the culture and context in which it took place' (p.45). It was racist because it mirrored the relative positions of 'Asian' and white boys in a society which is hierarchically ordered in terms of 'race'. What the panellists were pointing to were the structural implications of constructions of 'race'. Importantly, part of this general context was the school itself. The following points provide some sense of this:

- Darren Coulburn had had a history of picking on smaller, 'Asian' boys prior to this specific incident.
- Ahmed Ullah had had a history of trying to help these smaller boys in such circumstances.
- Darren Coulburn's behaviour was very much part of a more general racist culture within the school – so much so that the Report points out that many teachers and students gave evidence which suggested that the conduct from which the incident arose was not at all unusual or, indeed, offensive; it was just part of school life (pp.140–4).
- The panellists also suggested that the gender culture of the school, and of society more generally, was reflected in the behaviour of both boys, in that masculinity tended to be equated with aggressiveness (p.125).
- When Darren Coulburn had knifed Ahmed Ullah he depersonalized him by calling him 'a Paki', thus making use of the system of racist language and symbolism. This state of relations among the pupils of the school was mapped on to a racially tense atmosphere among the teaching staff of the school – racist jokes and comments 'permeated the whole school' (p.171).

It was such a situation as this that the head teacher – a Dr Gough – had been appointed to try to sort out in 1982. Upon his arrival in post he immediately instituted the new directive from the LEA to abolish corporal punishment and started to encourage student-centred teaching methods in place of more traditional ones. However, he also found that staff morale was low, that there were sharp tensions between racial groups on the two sites of the school, and that the management team set up to deal with all the issues was too small to undertake the task effectively (p.169). Given this, anti-racist policies were introduced:

- In 1982 a working party was established to begin the task of drafting the anti-racist policies. This draft was distributed to all staff in the spring of 1983 and after discussion this was amended to a second version distributed in the summer of that year (pp.172–3).

- In 1985, in accordance with the policy of the LEA, a racist incident log book was instituted. By the autumn of 1986 further guidelines on the identification of racist incidents and proposals for a more adequate recording system were circulated to staff and *black but not white parents*. This was revised in January 1987 (p.174).

- By 1985 there was less resistance, on the part of staff at the school, to the introduction of anti-racist policies and, as awareness about the complexities of the issues increased, some dissatisfaction with the limitations of the earlier document were expressed. These dissatisfactions centred on home–school liaison, pastoral care, the teaching of English as a second language, institutional racism in the school's own practices, and the lack of involvement of *black* students and *black* parents in the formulation of the original document (p.174).

- Following this, in the autumn of 1986 there was a proposal for the production of a new anti-racist policy for the school. Once drawn up this was to be circulated '*to black parents for discussion, whilst white parents were not involved*' (p.174).

- An Ethnic Minority Advisory Group was also set up. The establishment of a group for black parents only 'caused concern and hostility. Rightly so, in our view' (p.177).

This decision was the result of the way in which the problem of racism in schools, and the constituencies with responsibility for challenging it, were constructed in the particular version of anti-racism instituted at Burnage. As the panellists of the inquiry were to write:

> To Dr Gough a pre-requisite for the whole community getting together … is the empowerment of black parents. Black parents, be it noted. *Not white and black parents. But only black parents.* He sees white parents entirely negatively, just wanting a piece of the action, being resistant to anti-racism, being the possible cause of their own alienation, being suspicious and being adequately consulted through monthly meetings of the Parent's Society. Since these issues are particularly important to black parents it is obvious that they should be consulted, as he [Dr Gough] told us, but he did not feel that there should always be joint meetings, in which *white* parents could take part, and he was totally resistant to any suggestion that the Ethnic Minority Advisory Group in Burnage might have been a mistake.

And that:

> The notion of 'community' as necessarily embracing the white community, and 'multi-cultural' as including the culture of white working class people appears to have been ignored …
>
> (The Burnage Report, 1989, pp.178–9, 181, emphasis added)

What does this case study tell us about the relation between policies and social constructions?

Summary

We can see from this consideration of the Burnage Report that the boundaries of 'race' were constructed by the inversion of the dominant meanings attributed to physical variation of bodies. Thus *whiteness* itself was constructed as the problem to be 'solved' by the 'anti-racist' policy, when this policy should instead have been directed at a system of structured inequalities around a notion of 'race' which needed to be addressed by people from all sections of the school community. In this case the associations of 'good' and 'bad' across a white/black divide were inverted so that all white people came to be constructed as 'bad'.

Following from this, racism was considered to be an issue for black people only, an idea premised on the implicit assumption that white people could not be anti-racist. This is, however, an ironic position to adopt since the chief architects of the anti-racist policy were the head teacher and his deputy, both of whom were white. There is an added implication of this approach which suggests that white *working-class* people (the school was generally understood as serving a working-class catchment area) cannot be anti-racist. In contrast, white middle-class people can be.

This had the inevitable consequence of excluding white people from being involved in evolving an ethos of anti-racism in the school. Yet, equally inevitably, this approach could do nothing to undermine the wider structure of racial exclusions found outside the school, a structure of which the school pupils were well aware, as evidenced in the incident in which Darren Coulburn makes an Asian boy stand and sit while he says 'sorry, master'.

Finally, this examination of the Burnage Report provides an illustration of the links between social policies and social constructions. It shows us that there is a two-way link between the construction of social difference, in this case 'racial' difference, and the policies aimed at responding to it; and that these policies will themselves help to construct social difference. What Burnage also illustrates is that the construction of racial difference can also result in exclusions of groups of people who do not have a history of being the 'victims' of such racialization.

In section 6.1 we look further at processes by which racial categories and boundaries are constructed: but in the context of two important changes or shifts. One of these changes is a shift in the institutional arrangements between central and local government which ensued after a key piece of legislation was passed by a Conservative government. The other is a conceptual shift in the markers around which processes of racialization occurred.

6   Conceptual break

We will begin with the conceptual shift first. So far in this chapter we have been working with the conceptual category of 'race', which we have understood as a socially constructed category. At times, however, we have also mentioned the word 'ethnicity' and have argued that the term 'ethnic minorities' had come to replace that of 'immigrant' as the most common way of constructing a racialized subject. How, then, are we to distinguish between the terms 'race' and 'ethnicity'? At one level this is not an easy task since the terms are often used interchangeably. More generally, however, 'ethnicity' tends to be used to refer to cultural differences – so that 'ethnic minorities' are defined by the assumed cultural difference they have from the majority. Logically this should mean that *all* groups of people – 'majority' as well as 'minority' – could be defined by their cultural practices.

ethnicity

ACTIVITY 3.7

Make a quick list of all those groups you would automatically include under the heading 'ethnic minority'.

COMMENT

It is likely that you will have included such groups as 'Asians', 'Africans', 'African-Caribbeans', 'Muslims' and 'Jews', for example. Did you also include such groups as 'white people' or 'the English'?

■ ■ ■

That the term 'ethnicity' is usually applied only to groups of people who are racialized because of their colour is illustrated in the work on welfare citizenship by two social scientists. In presenting their findings they give brief details of the sample survey and do so in terms of the number who were 'white', 'black' (African-Caribbean) and 'Asian' (in fact none of the sample were 'Asian'), and in terms of gender. Yet, when they go on to consider the influence of 'diversity and difference' on their findings, under the section apparently dealing with 'ethnicity' they write: 'Our capacity to comment on the influence of ethnicity is hampered by our failure to include in the sample representatives of any Asian communities' (Dean and Melrose, 1996, p.27).

   If 'ethnicity' is simply a word which denotes 'culture', then this is a surprising statement to make, since they could have attempted to look at the influence of cultural differences between African-Caribbean participants in the sample and their 'white' counterparts. Their failure to do so reflects the common association of ethnicity with 'non-whiteness'. It also suggests that the term ethnicity connotes forms of boundary formation in which a normalized population (in this case 'white' people) is constructed as the group against which difference is defined.

   For this reason we will utilize the approach adopted by Barth (1969, p.300) and say that 'ethnicity' refers to the processes by which an ethnic 'boundary defines the group, [and] not the cultural stuff that it encloses'. In this sense the construction of ethnic groups and the ascription of people to them is a form of social organization. For our purposes what is of special importance is the point Barth made that 'culture' is not the defining feature of ethnicity and therefore should not be taken as the starting-point for identifying and analysing ethnic groups. Instead, identification and analysis of ethnicity requires recognition of three factors:

1   That ethnic groups are one way of organizing interaction between social actors who have been ascribed to, and identify with, a certain 'ethnic' category.

2   That ethnic boundaries are constructed in a social context.

3   That what is to be analysed are the social processes which generate and maintain these boundaries.

This means that attention is drawn to the boundaries or borders between groups and not to the factors which are assumed to be contained within these boundaries. So, for example, in the contemporary British context we would look at the wider social processes which lead to people being defined and identifying as, for instance, 'Asian', 'white', 'English', 'Welsh', 'black', 'Caribbean' or 'African'. We would not be looking at systems of marriage, or child-rearing, or cooking habits and tasks as the means by which to define ethnic belonging.

What does all this imply for the distinction between 'race' and 'ethnicity'? For our purposes there are three main issues:

1   First, it suggests that different signs or markers are used to indicate difference. For 'race' the signs are derived from physical variation. For 'ethnicity' the signs are derived from assumptions about cultural variation.

2   Second, it suggests that, because in the UK today 'colour' and other bodily variations are taken as an indicator of the existence of cultural variation, 'ethnicity' and 'race' are often used to stand for each other, which is why 'the ethnic communities' are most often associated with the 'non-white' populations in the UK.

3   Third, it suggests that both 'race' and 'ethnicity' are means of constructing social categories which then help to organize the social relations which characterize the UK today.

The following section illustrates the shift to 'ethnicity' as the major way of constructing racialized subjects and systems of 'racial' subordinations and exclusions.

6.1   'Race' and education after the Education Reform Act 1988: the changed institutional and legislative context

All the preceding events took place in the context of a specific organization of compulsory education which was laid down by the 1944 Education Act. Apart from setting out the division of secondary education into grammar, technical and secondary modern schools, the Act also established four main constituencies with overlapping responsibilities in the operation of state education: central government, local education authorities, parents and teachers.

The head teacher had a considerable degree of autonomy in how the school was run and it was precisely this structural decentralization which created the space for the adoption and implementation of anti-racist and multicultural policies in individual LEAs and individual schools (Ball and Troyna, 1989). But it was also the tensions which arose between some or all of these constituencies which gave rise to some of the most explicit forms of racialized exclusions. The examples of 'bussing' and Burnage illustrate well the shifting complexities of this process.

This structure remained basically intact until the 1988 Education Reform Act, which altered the balance between the four constituent parties of central and local government, parents and teachers. A major impact of this has been an increase in the relative power of the centre, either in the form of the Department of Education and Employment or in the form of quangos which are placed outside the forms of electoral accountability.

The mechanisms for the change were the introduction of a national curriculum, dictated by central government; the introduction of local management of schools; and the increase in 'parental choice', expressed through open enrolment and the potential to 'opt out' of LEA control. Together these provided a new framework in which education was to be delivered, administered and financed and in so doing it weakened the power of the local authority in education. These mechanisms gave rise to two countervailing trends which undermined and/or bypassed local authority power and control in this area – one centralizing, achieved through the introduction of a national curriculum; the other decentralizing, achieved through the other changes mentioned above. Macey (1992) has pointed to the implications of these trends:

> The imposition of a National Curriculum comprising 80% of the school timetable and the regular (standardised) assessment of pupil attainment will severely curtail teacher autonomy in terms of both curriculum content and teaching style, and the demand for teacher accountability via publication of pupil attainment will exert further pressure towards formal, didactic teaching techniques. Parental choice, encompassing open enrolment and 'opting out' of local education authority (LEA) control, has acute pedagogical and social implications and may exacerbate the trend towards racially segregated schools ... Opting out, which gives schools complete independence from LEA control and enables them to change their basic educational character, may further extend class, gender, religious and racial divisions in society ... Local management of schools (LMS) will significantly constrain the scope of LEAs to respond to local needs and could have a massive negative impact on already high levels of inequality, particularly in areas which have high concentrations of ethnic minority pupils.
>
> (Macey, 1992, pp.125–6)

The context for these changes was the general hostility of the Thatcher governments (1979–1982, 1982–1987, 1988–1990) and those of her successor, John Major (1990–1992, 1992–1997), to what was known as the Beveridge welfare state (for a detailed examination of these changes see **Hughes and Lewis, 1998**). Part of this hostility included a deep antagonism to the general multicultural ethos enshrined in the government reports of Rampton and Swann (Department of Education and Science, 1985). Ironically, however, this antagonism, like that of Swann, had at its centre a concern to achieve a socially, culturally and morally cohesive UK, which was deemed to have been eroded. In other words, just as in earlier national education policy, a particular vision of 'the British nation' was central to the 1988 education reforms. The national curriculum was to be the means by which the process of erosion of the British national identity might be stopped, as Kenneth Baker made clear when Secretary of State for Education in 1987:

> there is so much distraction, variety and uncertainty in the modern world that in our country today our children are in danger of losing any sense at all of a common culture and a common heritage. The cohesive role of the national curriculum will provide our society with a greater sense of identity.
>
> (Baker, 1987, para. 7)

The implication of this was also made clear by Baker when he made it known that funding for in-service training for teachers on matters of multicultural education was no longer to be a priority in national budgets for such training (reported in *The Guardian*, 16 August 1988), undermining the 'pursuit for equality' and ensuring that 'education has increasingly become defined and confined by central government' (Ball and Troyna, 1989, p.26).

It was not, however, just from politicians that the hostility to multicultural (in the form of the Swann Report) or anti-racist (in the form of the Institute of Race Relations evidence to the Rampton Committee) was to be heard. Along with sustained attacks on the content and methods of these pedagogic approaches in many newspapers during the 1980s, opposition was voiced from commentators, such as Geoffrey Partington (1984; 1985), educational practitioners, such as Ray Honeyford (1982; 1984; 1988), and philosophers, such as Roger Scruton (in *The Times*, 17 January 1984 and 16 April 1985) who were partisan to New Right or neo-Conservative thinking. Together these authors argued that:

- Multicultural and/or anti-racist education resulted in white children being disadvantaged because of the recognition of cultural diversity in school environments.
- This was in part the result of an 'inverted racism' which meant that Caribbean and south Asian children, and their assumed cultural backgrounds, were being privileged.
- Multicultural education confused education with propaganda.
- The patterns of under-achievement for some pupils from 'ethnic minority' backgrounds was a result of lack of support for the school and its values on the part of the parents of these children and of multicultural education itself.
- Multicultural and/or anti-racist education contributed to the emergence of social and political disintegration.

The effect of these arguments was to construct black pupils as outside the 'British nation' and so to reinforce processes of racialized differentiation and 'Othering'. The 'problem' was not envisaged as one of systemic racism and the exclusions to which this gives rise, but rather the 'hysterical political temperament of the Indian sub-continent' and the 'influential group of black intellectuals of aggressive disposition, who know little of the British traditions of understatement, civilized discourse and respect for reason' (Honeyford, 1984, pp.31–2).

If this was indicative of a shift in approach to multicultural education by the ruling power bloc, it was also mapped on to a realignment in the balance of power among the four main constituencies which were central to the 1944 structure of compulsory education. Thus the effect of the 1988 Education Reform Act was in part to shift power away from the LEA and towards parents, who, through 'opt out' and the local management of schools, could reinforce tendencies towards 'racial' and/or ethnic segregation in schools. Indeed, part of the rhetoric of some of the New Right thinkers on education was precisely to construct multicultural education as a professionally imposed system of education which went against the wishes of the majority of parents (Honeyford, 1988, pp.89–92). In this context any white parents who claimed dissatisfaction with the schooling their children were receiving, on the grounds of an imposed multicultural curriculum, were met with great applause by some sections of both the media and the intellectual establishment. We can see this clearly in the case of Headfield Junior School in Dewsbury, West Yorkshire.

The majority of pupils at this school were of south Asian descent and in August 1987 the parents of 26 white children refused to send their children to this school for this reason. The parents stated that they wanted their children to attend another school where the intake was mostly white, arguing that their concern was not 'racial' but cultural (or 'ethnic') and centred on the celebration of Muslim festivals in Headfield. As a result of the purported Muslim orientation of Headfield the parents said that Christmas was not celebrated, a claim vigorously denied by the school and the LEA, both of which pointed out that the school was in fact a Church of England school, with Christian assemblies each morning. Despite this:

> the language used in much of the press coverage lent support to the parents' cause. They were portrayed as 'rebels' fighting for a good education for 'weeping children' against an uncaring education authority and school which refused to accept them. At the same time the black pupils at Headfield were always portrayed as 'Asian', even though most of them were British born, and often this was contrasted with 'English', which meant 'white'.
>
> (Gordon and Rosenberg, 1989, pp.45–6)

The period leading up to the passing of the Education Reform Act in 1988 was, then, a time when the needs for and benefits of multicultural and anti-racist educational practice were increasingly challenged. Those challenges which emerged from the New Right became enshrined in the Act, together with an explicit promotion of what were called 'British values' and 'British culture'. In so doing, those defined as 'ethnic minority' were constructed as *in* but not *of* the nation and thus racialized exclusions were perpetuated. As we have seen, this just marked a new stage in a continuous but uneven process of such racializing practices within education – it is, however, important to grasp the changes in and subtleties of processes of racial or ethnic boundary formation. Activity 3.8 should help with this.

Ray Honeyford, a former head teacher, came to some prominence in the early to mid 1980s when, after a series of articles in the *Times Educational Supplement* and the *Salisbury Review*, his views on multicultural and anti-racist education brought him into conflict with some black parents and the LEA which employed him. This conflict led to his resignation in 1985 from his post as head teacher at a school in Bradford which had a large number of pupils of south Asian descent. We are considering the approach of Honeyford at some length, not because he himself had an enduring influence, but rather because he reflected the shift to 'ethnicity' as the prime marker of 'racial' difference which characterized the late 1980s and 1990s. In the introduction to his book *Integration or Disintegration?*, Honeyford reiterated his much-stated claim that his concern was for the education of *all* children, that he felt all children were being let down by the pursuit of a multicultural curriculum, and that he:

was also worried about the manifestly tendentious view of British history, institutions and traditions that the mandatory [teaching] documents contained. Perhaps most telling of all, my objection was to the constant suggestion that all white people, and only white people, are 'racist', and could only expiate their guilt by supporting the multicultural/anti-racist bandwagon. I could not see how the transmission of this manifestly questionable, not to say offensive, allegation to children could possibly augur well for future race relations.

(Honeyford, 1988, pp.2–3)

His project, then, is one aimed at promoting what he calls a 'non-racist' position, which is, he believes, 'the position of the great majority of my fellow-countrymen' (Honeyford, 1988, p.ix).

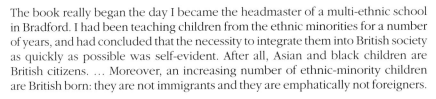

ACTIVITY 3.8

Now work through Extract 3.6, taken from later in Honeyford's book *Integration or Disintegration?: Towards a Non-Racist Society*. As you do so, consider the following questions:

1   What view of British society is portrayed in the extract?

2   Are 'ethnic minority' cultures portrayed as being *of* Britain?

3   Is there any notion that power structures the relations between diverse ethnic groups?

4   What consequence are advocacy and promotion of cultural pluralism said to have for social and political cohesion?

Extract 3.6 Honeyford: 'Integration or disintegration?'

The book really began the day I became the headmaster of a multi-ethnic school in Bradford. I had been teaching children from the ethnic minorities for a number of years, and had concluded that the necessity to integrate them into British society as quickly as possible was self-evident. After all, Asian and black children are British citizens. ... Moreover, an increasing number of ethnic-minority children are British born: they are not immigrants and they are emphatically not foreigners. ...

Underlying much multi-ethnic rhetoric is the notion that unless ethnic-minority cultures are preserved and transmitted by the schools they will wither and die. This is to fly in the face of the evidence. The Irish, Jews and central Europeans are all examples of successful immigrant communities which have kept their original cultures alive and flourishing, without any attempt to see them self-consciously fostered in the state schools. Moreover, there is no evidence for public support for the state to promote foreign cultures in the schools. In truth, cultures can only live and continue in the social context in which they are practised. Can they be tagged onto, or absorbed into, existing cultures by government decree? How many teachers, or educational experts, does Britain have capable of mastering all the minority cultures that now exist so as to create a genuinely imported and representative cultural mosaic as the basis for the school curriculum? Perhaps the new cross-cultural curricula are to be fashioned by teams of experts from the different communities. One wonders how the Moslem and Hindu representatives on such a committee might wish to see the partition of India taught, or how slavery should be conveyed assuming a debate between a Jamaican and English academic ... .

The claim that established school curricula are narrowly Anglo-Saxon … is questionable. The briefest look at any typical school curriculum will indicate a mosaic of influences. The Bible, for instance, is an essentially foreign influence taken over from the Jews. Literature and science have roots in Greek and Roman experience. Our mathematics has been influenced by Arabic notions imported after the Crusades. Geography syllabuses have always included the study of far-away places and exotic peoples. Our greatest dramatist provides experience of cultures and characters that lie far beyond the everyday life of English people – consider *Julius Caesar, Othello, The Merchant of Venice* and *Hamlet,* and all that they represent in the way of other cultures and thought … Art teaching has included exotic influence for generations, including the art of Africa, India, and the Near East, … and no one can accuse the English language of narrowness and rigidity; it is an amalgam of an astonishing range of influences. …

This openness to the world ought not to surprise us. The historic role of Britons as seafarers, explorers and empire-builders has encouraged immensely powerful cross-cultural forces. …

Multi-ethnic advocacy inevitably tends towards demands for the community language to be both on the curriculum and the medium of instruction …

Now there undoubtedly is a case for community languages such as Punjabi, Urdu, Pushtu or Gujerati to be placed on the curriculum where there is parental demand and the resources are available. There are, however, obvious dangers. … [I]f we allow one community language as a school subject then we set a precedent for a demand for *all* such languages to be taught … If we accept only certain languages for inclusion, then we risk jealousy and resentment from those whose languages are not selected. … The virtue of confining language teaching to the traditional ones (for example, French, German, Spanish, etc.) is that they are not associated with minority groups living in Britain, so there can be no inter-racial squabbling between different minority groups. Of course, precisely the same objections can be made of the multi-ethnic curriculum in general – whose cultures ought it to reflect …? …

Advocates of a multi-ethnic curriculum often appear unaware of the relationship between the formal educational process and the maintenance of social and political cohesion. Reflecting a diversity of cultural styles may appear to be both enriching and humane and, in principle, eminently defensible. What, however, of its predictable, consequential effects? Are established social institutions based on the principle of cultural pluralism, or do they proceed on the basis of a common public culture, with minority lifestyles being an essential, but private, matter? Do they not, for instance, assume a common, national language and access to a common set of presuppositions about procedures and beliefs in the management of human needs? Is there not, for instance, an essentially Western, capitalist, mixed economy to which everyone has access either as worker, manager or investor? … How far can respect for diversity by the state through the schools system go, before the process becomes divisive?

(Honeyford, 1988, pp.1, 88, 84–5, 85–6, 88–9)

COMMENT

In many ways it is difficult to unpack or 'deconstruct' the discourses of 'race' and/or 'ethnicity' which are contained within this extract. However, it is possible to see the following when working through it.

'Britain' was presented as being both *historically* made up of a 'mosaic of influences' and based on a 'common public culture' with a 'common set of presuppositions' in the *late 1980s* when Honeyford was writing. In this way, being *of* Britain is not the same as being *in* Britain and the Britain of today is not the same as that of yesterday. Thus contemporary British society is made up of a *majority of Britons who share these presuppositions*, and a *minority of culturally diverse people whose presuppositions are a 'private matter'*. Within the 'British' majority *class or status position is not about division or exclusion from society*, since 'worker, manager, or investor' has access to the mixed economy.

This portrayal of Britain, then, necessarily constructs *those defined as 'ethnic minority cultures' as different from and outside the 'nation'* in terms of its ethnic roots. But because they are physically in Britain *potential antagonisms among them must be prevented by the cohesive force of the English language*. Public recognition and support for their cultural habits and languages must not be forthcoming otherwise these antagonisms will be able to flourish. It is also in the portrayal of 'ethnic minorities' as potentially in conflict with one another that we can see how the author constructs a hard boundary between these groups and 'the British'. For it is only the minority groups which are presented as potentially disruptive to British society. It is the Muslim and the Hindu, the Punjabi speaker or their Gujerati-speaking counterpart who is potentially divisive. We also see hard boundaries being constructed around notions of 'race' (and nationality) in the suggestion that a Jamaican and an English academic could not agree about how to teach the history of British slavery and the Atlantic slave trade.

Yet despite this construction of racial and ethnic divides, Honeyford *avoids any suggestion that these divisions are in some way structured in and through relations of power*. Britain's historical 'openness to the world', the 'exotic influences', and the study of 'exotic peoples' are all referred to as if this openness, influence and study occurred in a system of equal relations. This is, of course, consistent with the portrayal of British society as equal in terms of class. Once Honeyford has presented Britain as historically forged out of a mosaic of ethnic influences and as a cohesive and equal society today, it is then easy for him to suggest that *public recognition and support of cultural diversity would be socially and politically divisive*.

These are some of the points evident in Extract 3.6. Compare them with the points that you came up with. Finally, given Honeyford's stated concern for *all* children, you should consider to what extent you think *all* children would feel equally valued. Would *you*, for example, feel valued and supported in a system of education organized with this view of cultural diversity?

■ ■ ■

7   Is being white enough?: racialization and the Irish in Britain

As we have worked through this chapter the 'subjects' of racial discourse have, in the main, been black or 'non-white' people. As a chapter on the social construction of 'race' this may appear 'natural', 'normal' or 'inevitable'.

Why might it appear 'natural' that a chapter on 'race' will be about black or 'non-white' people?

There were, however, two places where white people were the focus of attention – in sections 1 and 2, where we considered the issue of the body, 'race' and place; and then again in section 5 when we considered the racial exclusions which were said to have occurred at Burnage High School.

Here we want to consider further the issue of 'race' and whiteness by thinking about processes of racialization and the Irish in Britain. Let us begin by reminding ourselves of what is meant by racialization. Earlier, I suggested that racialization was a process comprising:

1   Specific groups of people are constructed as a 'type' in reference to a limited number of selected physical or cultural features.

2   Their actual or assumed behaviour, abilities and values are then 'explained' by reference to those selected features.

It is possible to see evidence of this process in relation to the Irish by comparing these two statements from the nineteenth century: 'The English people are naturally industrious ... now of all the Celtic tribes, famous everywhere for their indolence and fickleness ... the Irish are admitted to be the most idle and the most fickle. They will not work if they can exist without it' (*Frazer's Magazine*, 1847, reprinted in Lebow, 1976, p.44). And this from Frederick Engels, friend and comrade of Karl Marx:

> These Irish workers pay only fourpence passage-money to get to England and they are often packed like cattle on the deck of the steamboat. ... The worst accommodation is good enough for them; they take no trouble with regard to their clothes which hang in tatters; they go barefoot. They live solely on potatoes and any money left over ... goes on drink. Such folk do not need high wages. The slums of all the big towns swarm with Irish. ... These faces are quite different from those of the Anglo-Saxon population and are easily recognisable. ... [T]he Irish have discovered ... the minimum of the means of life ... [and have] brought with them filth and intemperance.
>
> (Engels, 1971, p.105)

These quotations, in their different ways, are clear examples of the social construction of the Irish as a category of people who are 'knowable' by assumed essential characteristics. By suggesting that these characteristics are also 'natural', they indicate as well the ways in which social constructions essentialize by naturalizing the social ascriptions tied to racializations.

One common form in which racializations present themselves is as stereotypes. As with black groups who are racialized, stereotypes of the Irish are not just a thing of the past and remain an active part of the process by which Irish people become known as a 'racial' type.

A popular form of racialization is via the joke.

Do you think that 'Irish jokes' are racist or racializing?

In Britain the 'Irish joke' has been a common way of racializing the Irish and of constructing a stereotyped Irish man or woman. In 1979, Edmund Leach, an English anthropologist, analysed a number of anti-Irish joke books and found that:

The prototype of the stage Irishmen … is not so much a figure of fun as an object of contempt merging into deep hostility. He is a drink-addicted moron, reared in the bog, who wears his rubber boots at all times, cannot read or write, and constantly reverses the logic of ordinary common-sense. His female counterpart shares the same qualities, except that she is sexually promiscuous, rather than perpetually drunk … The ethnic element in 'Irish' jokes is thus blatantly racist.

(Leach, 1979, pp.viii–ix)

This brief exploration clearly illustrates the ways in which a white group is racialized. Thus when we talk about the social construction of 'race' we are referring not only to the construction of 'non-white' peoples, but to all people. Where racial categorization is a feature of social organization, white people as well as 'non-white' are also racially categorized. This is not always easy to see because, when looking at 'race', we tend to look at the subordinated or marginalized groups and not at the dominant or normalized ones, and to assume that all white people are constructed as dominant. Thus studies of 'race' and ethnicity in the UK today do not tend to be about the white populations of England, Wales, Scotland and Northern Ireland and therefore we do not see how 'racial' and ethnic subordinations are constructed among them.

For the Irish in Britain the complexities of what is seen and what is hidden from view by dominant approaches to 'race' are quite profound. As an 'ethnic group' – that is, as 'the Irish' – they are, as we have seen, subject to racialization. However, because they are (in the main) white, and because 'race' or 'ethnicity' is supposed to be about black people, the ways in which this racialization subordinates them and affects their material circumstances is often hidden from view. In other words, it is relatively easy to see the ways in which the Irish in contemporary Britain are *discursively* constructed as racial subjects but less easy to see how these constructions solidify in ways which affect their structural position. We do, however, have some evidence of the ways in which the racialization of the Irish affects their experience of housing and health.

In terms of housing the Irish have a profile near to that of the racialized group most disadvantaged in terms of housing: that is, Bangladeshis. Both groups have the lowest share of owner occupation – at 34 per cent for Irish and 32 per cent for Bangladeshis; in London these groups are most likely to be in accommodation condemned as unfit or as lacking or sharing basic amenities (London Borough of Haringey, 1992). The Irish are also over-represented in homeless figures (CARA, 1988) and a survey of the Irish community's service needs carried out in 1993 showed that 29 per cent of the sample lived in short-term insecure housing, whilst 17 per cent were reported as homeless, especially if they were men in the under-25 age group (Kowarzik, 1994).

Data on mortality and health also provide evidence of the disadvantaged social location of the Irish in Britain. One particularly stark factor is that of mortality rates. As one report noted on the basis of several studies: 'analysis of longitudinal census data indicates that the Irish now have the highest standardized mortality rates of all groups in Britain. The Irish are the only migrant group whose life expectancy worsens upon arrival in Britain' (London Borough of Haringey, 1992, p.5). Moreover, figures from the 1993 Labour Force Survey show that 20 per cent of Irish-born people of working age, living in Britain, had a health problem or disability which limited their ability to work. The comparable figure for the rest of the population was 14 per cent (Woolford, 1994).

Summary

Data such as these are often taken as indicative of discrimination when applied to those populations termed 'ethnic minorities'. In relation to the Irish, however, a similar association is obscured from view as the dominant common sense links 'race' and discrimination to 'non-white' groups only.

In this section we have suggested that a racially structured society will mean that *all* people are racialized. We have also suggested that some groups will experience discrimination as a result of racialization even though they are 'white'. Finally, we have given some very brief indications of this in relation to the Irish in Britain.

8 Conclusion

In this chapter we have considered ways in which that most personal of things – the body – becomes situated in systems of meaning which both reflect *past* and present social relations and also structure experience. In particular, we have looked at the links between the racial marking of bodies and social exclusions.

Most importantly we suggested that 'racial groups' are socially constructed. Such social constructions have 'real life' effects in that they help to organize the social interactions between individuals and groups. That is, they help organize and give meaning to the interactions between people who are 'known' as 'racial' or 'ethnic' and those who are not known in this way. In the UK today this is most commonly understood as reflecting the divide between 'black' and 'white'. However, an important aspect of the argument in this chapter has been that *all* groups are racialized – some, however, experience this racialization *ex*plicitly, while others – mainly those defined as 'white' – experience it *im*plicitly.

Like the social construction of other forms of 'difference', the construction of 'race' and ethnicity will have a profound influence on the formation and implementation of social policies. We have looked at ways in which social policies carry the traces of, *and* rework, such social constructions and so reproduce the processes of racial inclusion and exclusion.

We have looked briefly at these connections in relation to immigration policy and the Irish experience of welfare. However, education provided the site for our extended exploration of the links between social policy and racial exclusions. What this allowed us to see was that the marking of social difference (in this case around notions of 'race' and ethnicity) – and the exclusions to which this gives rise – is never a once-and-for-all event. It is instead a *process* which requires a continual reworking if it is to be maintained. By looking at different 'moments' in official education policy we were able to see how 'race' and ethnicity were continually reconceptualized in the attempt to find appropriate forms of education for a multiracial and multi-ethnic population. We also saw that the construction of difference is always accompanied by forms of resistance and contestation and suggested that these contestations may also result in exclusions.

Further reading

A useful collection of historical and contemporary articles on ethnicity can be found in Sollars (1996). These articles are helpful for charting the different and conflicting ways in which ethnicity as a concept is defined and used. A feminist analysis of the intersections between gender, 'race' and class in the organization of global and national relations is given in Eisenstein (1996). This is useful for those interested in developing their understanding of the social construction of the body. Mercer (1994) has compiled a collection of essays mapping the development and context of black British identities since the 1960s. This is especially useful for those wishing to explore further the social construction of forms of ethnic belonging. Invaluable for its discussion of the concepts of 'race', racialization and ethnicity is *Racialized Boundaries* by Anthias and Yuval-Davis (1992) which links these concepts to issues of class and gender and the anti-racist struggle in the UK. Finally, two pamphlets pertaining to the racialization of Irish people in Britain: Curtis (1984) charts the historical roots of this racialization, and Hazelkorn (1990) offers a clear introduction to the socio-economic position of the Irish in Britain.

References

Anderson, B. (1983) *Imagined Communities*, London, Verso.

Anthias, F. and Yuval-Davis, N. (in association with H. Cains) (1992) *Racialized Boundaries*, London, Routledge.

Baker, K. (1987) Speech given at Manchester University, 17 September, London, HMSO.

Ball, W. and Troyna, B. (1989) 'The dawn of a new era? The Education Reform Act, "race" and LEAs', *Educational Management and Administration*, no.17, pp.23–31.

Barth, F. (1969) 'Introduction to ethnic groups and boundaries', in Sollars (1996).

Bevan, V. (1986) *The Development of British Immigration Law*, London, Croom Helm.

Bolton, E.J. (1979) 'Education in a multi-racial society', *Trends in Education*, Winter, pp.3–7.

Bruce-Pratt, M. (1988) 'Identity: skin, blood, heart', in Crowley, H. and Himmelweit, S. (eds) (1992) *Knowing Women*, Cambridge, Polity Press in association with The Open University.

Butler, J. (1993) *Bodies that Matter*, New York and London, Routledge.

Campaign Against Racism and Fascism, and Southall Rights (1981) *Birth of a Black Community*, London, Institute of Race Relations.

CARA (1988) *Irish Homelessness: The Hidden Dimension, A Strategy for Change*, London, Irish Housing Association Ltd.

Commonwealth Immigrants Advisory Council (1964) Second Report, London, HMSO.

Curtis, L. (1984) *Nothing But the Same Old Story: The Roots of Anti-Irish Racism*, Information on Ireland, London.

Dean, H. and Melrose, M. (1996) 'Unravelling citizenship: the significance of social security fraud', *Critical Social Policy*, vol.16, no.3, pp.3–31.

Department of Education and Science (1965) *The Education of Immigrants*, London, HMSO.

Department of Education and Science (1985) *Education for All*, The Report of the Committee of Inquiry into the Education of Children from Ethnic Minority Groups, chaired by Lord Swann (The Swann Report), Cmnd 9453, London, HMSO.

Eisenstein, Z. (1996) *Hatreds*, New York and London, Routledge.

Engels, F. (1971) *The Condition of the Working Class in England* (trans. and ed. W.O. Henderson and W.T. Chaloner), Oxford, Blackwell.

Faist, T. (1995) *Social Citizenship for Whom?: Young Turks in Germany and Mexican Americans in the USA*, Aldershot, Avebury.

Fryer, P. (1984) *Staying Power*, London, Pluto.

Gordon, P. and Klug, F. (1985) *British Immigration Control: A Brief Guide*, London, Runnymede Trust.

Gordon, P. and Rosenberg, D. (1989) *Daily Racism: The Press and Black People in Britain*, London, The Runnymede Trust.

Gurney, J. (ed.) (1993) *Ethnic Minorities Benefits Handbook*, Leeds, Chapeltown Law Centre.

Hall, S. and Held, D. (1989) 'Left and rights', *Marxism Today*, June, pp.16–23.

Hazelkorn, E. (1990) *Irish Immigrants Today: A Socio-Economic Profile of Comtemporary Irish Emigrants and Immigrants in the UK*, London, PNL Press, University of North London.

Hickman, M. (1998) 'Education for "minorities": the Irish in Britain', in Lewis, G. (ed.) *Forming Nation, Framing Welfare*, London, Routledge in association with The Open University.

Honeyford, R. (1982) 'Multiracial myths?', *Times Educational Supplement*, 19 November, p.12.

Honeyford, R. (1984) 'Education and race – an alternative view', *Salisbury Review*, no.6, pp.30–2.

Honeyford, R. (1988) *Integration or Disintegration?: Towards a Non-Racist Society*, London, The Claridge Press.

Hughes, G. and Lewis, G. (eds) (1998) *Unsettling Welfare: The Reconstruction of Social Policy*, London, Routledge in association with The Open University.

Institute of Race Relations (1980) 'Anti-racist not multicultural education: IRR statement to the Rampton Committee on Education', *Race & Class*, vol.XXII, no.1, pp.81–3.

Jenkins, R. (1966) Address given by the Home Secretary to Voluntary Liaison Committees, London, NCCI.

Kearney, H. (1995) *The British Isles: A Story of Four Nations*, Cambridge, Cambridge University Press.

Kowarzik, U. (1994) *Developing a Community Response: The Service Needs of the Irish Community in Britain*, commissioned by The Action Group for Irish Youth and the Federation of Irish Societies.

Leach, E. (1979) 'The official Irish jokesters', *New Society*, 20–27 December, pp.vii–ix.

Lebow, R.N. (1976) 'White Britain and black Ireland: the influence of stereotypes on colonial policy', Philadelphia, MA, Institute for the Study of Human Issues.

Levitas, R. (1996) 'The concept of social exclusion and the new Durkheimian hegemony', *Critical Social Policy*, vol.16, no.1, pp.5–20.

Lewis, G. (1985) 'From deepest Kilburn', in Heron, L. (ed.) *Truth, Dare or Promise: Girls Growing Up in the Fifties*, London, Virago.

Lister, R. (1990) *The Exclusive Society: Citizenship and the Poor*, London, Child Poverty Action Group.

London Borough of Haringey (1992) *Equal Opportunities: The Irish Dimension*, London, Haringey Council.

Macey, M. (1992) 'The 1988 Education Reform Act: has multicultural education any future?', *British Journal of the Sociology of Education*, vol.13, no.1, pp.125–30.

Marshall, T.H. (1950) *Citizenship and Social Class*, Cambridge, Cambridge University Press.

Mercer, K. (1993) '1968: periodising politics and identity', in Mercer (1994).

Mercer, K. (1994) *Welcome to the Jungle: New Positions in Black Cultural Studies*, London, Routledge.

Mullard, C. (1982) 'Multiracial education in Britain: from assimilation to cultural pluralism', in Tierney, J. *et al.* (eds) *Race, Migration and Schooling*, New York, Holt.

OFSTED (1996) *Recent Research on the Achievement of Ethnic Minority Pupils* (prepared by D. Gillborn and C. Gipps), London, HMSO.

Partington, G. (1984) 'Race, sex and class in inner London', *Salisbury Review*, no.7, pp.33–7.

Partington, G. (1985) 'The same or different? Curricular implications of feminism and multiculturalism', *Journal of Curriculum Studies*, vol.17, no.3, pp.275–92.

Rattansi, A. (1992) 'Changing the subject? Racism, culture and education', in Donald, J. and Rattansi, A. (eds) *Race: Culture and Difference*, London, Sage.

Sollars, W. (ed.) (1996) *Theories of Ethnicity*, Basingstoke, Macmillan.

The Burnage Report (1989) *Murder in the Playground*, London, Longsight Press.

The Open University (1978) E361 *Education and the Urban Environment*, Block V *Race and Education*, Units 12 and 13, *Race, Children and Cities*, Milton Keynes, The Open University.

Townsend, H.E.R. (1971) *Immigrant Pupils in England: The LFA Response*, Slough, NFER.

Turner, B. (1996) *The Body and Society*, Oxford, Blackwell.

Woolford, C. (1994) 'Irish nationals in the British labour market', *Employment Gazette*, January, pp.23–8.

CHAPTER 4

Abnormal, Unnatural and Immoral? The Social Construction of Sexualities

by Esther Saraga

Contents

1   Introduction

In this chapter we shall explore social constructionism in relation to a further aspect of social difference, namely sexuality. Sexuality is a particularly interesting area to consider as it seems to be one of the most obviously natural aspects of human life, clearly rooted in our biological make-up. However, as you know from discussions in earlier chapters, it is precisely in relation to what seems most obvious that we need to develop the greatest scepticism, and question the taken-for-granted assumptions underlying what are thought of as 'common-sense' views. As we do this in relation to sexuality, we shall explore many of the central themes of this book that were identified in Chapter 1.

■   Section 2 examines dominant definitions of sexuality within 'common senses' and within a range of written extracts. Our major concern is to see how sexuality is constructed in terms of the 'natural' and the 'normal'. We shall explore the consequences of these constructions for creating particular subject positions, and for identifying particular forms of sexuality as deviant and as social problems which need to be controlled or hidden.

■   Section 3 explores two competing perspectives on sexuality, essentialism and social constructionism, and shows the historical development of social constructionism as a challenge to essentialism.

■   Section 4 is an introduction to the case studies examined in the next two sections.

■   Sections 5 and 6 explore further the ideas raised in the chapter through two case studies (on prostitution and homosexuality) which allow us to see historical continuities and changes in the way these issues have been socially constructed, and their very real consequences for people's lives.

As with Chapters 2 and 3, our primary concern is to examine social constructionist approaches within social science. As an account of ideas and issues concerned with sexuality, it is necessarily selective and incomplete. As you read the chapter it would be helpful to note those features which are similar to the explorations of disability and 'race', and those which are distinctive to a discussion of sexuality.

2   Questions of definition: what is sexuality?

2.1   Common senses

Let us start by considering the narrower term 'sex', a word used frequently in everyday language in many different contexts. Most commonly it refers to:

1   biological sex, a distinction between two *categories of people*, defined as 'female' or 'male' in terms of particular characteristics of their bodies; and

2   'having sex', a description of *physical activities*, generally thought of as heterosexual intercourse, linked to biological processes of reproduction.

Reflecting on these two common understandings of 'sex', we see that they are not quite so straightforward. First, the distinction between two 'biological sexes' is complicated by the existence of some people not easily categorized by their external genitalia (described as hermaphrodites), and of others who feel their anatomical body is out of line with their subjective sense of being male or female (described as transsexuals). The categories male and female do not therefore simply describe biological features of bodies. Moreover, when we identify someone as 'male' or 'female', it is very rarely based on their bodily features, but on other characteristics such as hair, clothes, behaviour and voice, all of which have social meanings, varying with factors like age, culture and 'race'. In order to distinguish between the apparently natural biological fact of 'sex', and the social and cultural characteristics of being male or female, the term gender is frequently used for the latter. We shall return in section 3.3 to some difficulties raised by this distinction. The important point here is to see that an apparently simple biological fact of nature is rather more complex.

gender

Second, in considering 'sex' as physical activities, we recognize that in most cases the goal of sexual activity is not reproduction. It may involve a range of different behaviours, with or without vaginal penetration, such as masturbation or looking at pornography; it may not involve two people; and the sexual activity may not be heterosexual. The need to broaden the definition poses a difficult question: what characteristics define a particular form of behaviour as 'sexual'? If we include fantasy and desire, which cannot be observed as behaviour; if we recognize that for some of us our sexuality is central to our sense of identity, or is used by others as a way of defining us; and if we acknowledge historical and cultural variations in sexual practices, identities and attitudes, the question of definition becomes very complex.

What is considered 'sexual' is not fixed. There is huge variation in the social meanings attached to it. Because of these ambiguities and complexities, and the many aspects of human experience that may be seen as 'sexual', we have used the broader term 'sexuality' in this chapter to encompass sexual practices, desires, identities and gender distinctions.

ACTIVITY 4.1

Before reading further, write down all the different meanings that 'sexuality' has for you.

COMMENT

You may have included some of the following ideas:

- Sexuality is about bodily sensations; 'having sex' is seen as spontaneous and instinctual, necessary to satisfy a biological 'need' or urge.
- Sexual practices are generally expected to be pleasurable, but they can also be used abusively, to coerce and harm others.
- Common senses see a particular form of sexual behaviour – heterosexual intercourse – as 'real sex' and hence the 'best' way to be sexual. It is seen as most natural, therefore normal and morally superior, and hence most satisfying.
- Other sexualities are therefore unnatural, abnormal and immoral.
- Sexuality as physical relationships is generally seen as a matter of private concern.
- Sex is commonly viewed as secret and largely invisible.
- Sexuality is seen to develop in puberty and is appropriate for mature adults; children are expected to be sexually innocent.

- Sex is associated with love, intimacy and desire, with attractiveness and 'fancying' others; there are dominant ideas on what constitutes attractiveness in any particular society, and these change historically.

- Sexual relationships are seen as qualitatively different from other kinds of relationships such as friendship.

- People differ in their sexuality; the most obvious differences are those assumed to exist between men and women.

- Sexuality is experienced subjectively; for each individual it can be a source of pleasure, anxiety, pain or abuse, and this may vary through our lifetime. Because it is seen as natural and biological, it is widely believed to be characteristic of our 'true selves' and to give us our identities.

- Since the 1980s, anxiety about HIV and AIDS, and constructions of AIDS as a 'gay plague', have had an impact on ideas about different kinds of sexual practices ('safer sex'), as well as on lesbian and gay communities.

■ ■ ■

You may have recognized some tensions and contradictions in these ideas. On the one hand sexuality is seen as the expression of a natural, biologically based drive. On the other hand, advice is offered in magazine articles and books on how to gain more satisfaction, and there are normative views on the morally best ways of being sexual (for example, monogamous heterosexuality within marriage). In the popular press, in particular, many sexualities are seen as both deviant and newsworthy, simultaneously condemned and the object of perpetual fascination. There may also be tensions between sex as 'pleasure' and sex as 'danger', between sex as something sought after or feared. As we have seen in earlier chapters, the consequences of defining particular forms of human behaviour and experience as natural is that by implication other forms are deemed unnatural, and hence problematic and often also morally dangerous. We shall be considering this in greater detail later in the chapter.

normative

Is sexuality a social issue?

Sexuality is not just a private matter. In contemporary Western industrialized societies, sex is around us all the time – it is used to entertain (in films and novels and on television), it is sold directly itself (prostitution, pornography, sex aids), and it is used to sell a wide range of other products (from hair spray to cars). One of the legacies of Freud's work is that sexuality is seen to pervade, most often unconsciously, all aspects of individual, social and cultural behaviour. Part of its power would seem to be the breaking of taboos, an involvement with something forbidden, secret or feared.

Although sexuality is publicly pervasive, people's sexual behaviour and practices are supposed to be secret and private. They can be difficult to talk about, and perhaps even to read and write about as part of academic study. Discussions of sex can arouse feelings of anxiety, disgust, curiosity and humour, as well as being a bit 'naughty'. In some contexts it becomes 'permissible' to talk about sex, for example during 'sex education' in schools, with a doctor or nurse in a family planning clinic, as a group of men in the pub, or among women on a 'girls' night out'. In each context there are particular shared meanings of 'sexuality'.

*Sexuality is used to sell a wide range of products.
Note the diverse representations of women's sexuality*

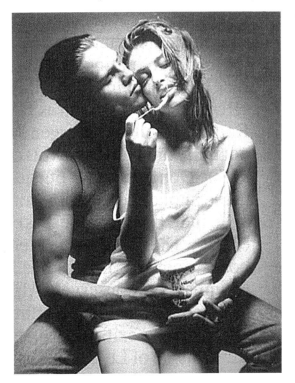

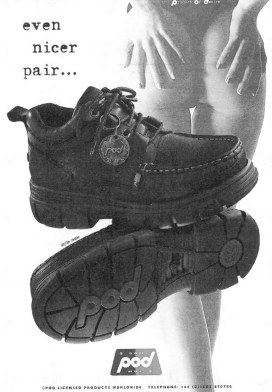

even
nicer
pair...

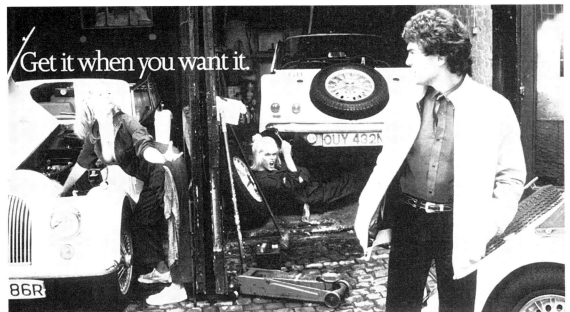

Sexuality may also be seen as a social problem, particularly if it challenges traditional morality and appears to threaten aspects of the social order, such as the purity of the nation, or the security of public spaces like the streets. In the 1990s, examples of social problems linked to sexuality might be lone-parent families, teenage pregnancies, high divorce rates, infertility treatments, abortion, prostitution, gays in the church and in the military, HIV and AIDS, child sexual abuse, paedophilia, the age of consent for male homosexuality, and lesbian and gay parenthood. You may well be able to add to this list.

2.2 Competing social constructions of sexuality

ACTIVITY 4.2

Some of the different ideas on sexuality that we have been exploring are reflected in writings about sexuality.

Read Extracts 4.1–4.4, bearing in mind the following questions:

1   How does each author define sexuality?

2   To what extent is sexuality seen as 'natural' or 'social'?

3   What ideas about 'normality' and 'deviance' can you identify?

Extract 4.1 Ellis: 'Psychology of sex'

Sex penetrates the whole person; a man's sexual constitution is a part of his general constitution. There is considerable truth in the dictum: 'A man is what his sex is' … we are all made up of various impulses, and the sexually normal man is often a man who holds in control some abnormal impulse. Yet in the main a man's sexual constitution is all-pervading, deep-rooted, permanent, in large measure congenital …

It was formerly taken for granted by all writers on the life of sex that there is but one pattern for that life, and that any straying from that one pattern was not 'normal'. This was assumed and never discussed … So far from there being only one pattern of sex-life, it would be nearer the truth to say that there are as many patterns as there are individuals … I have sought to make clear that here, as elsewhere in nature, we have to admit a wide limit of variation within the normal range …

In order to remain within the normal range, all variations must at some point include the procreative end for which sex exists. To exclude procreation is perfectly legitimate, and under some circumstances morally imperative. But sexual activities entirely and by preference outside the range in which procreation is possible may fairly be considered abnormal; they are deviations.

Sexual deviations were formerly called 'perversions'. That word arose at a time when sexual anomalies were universally regarded as sins or crimes, at the least as vices. It is still used by those whose ideas are rooted in traditions of the past which they cannot outgrow. In earlier years I have myself used it, though under protest, and with explanations of what I thereby meant. I now realize that … the time has come to avoid the word, so far as possible, altogether … it dates from days anterior to the scientific and medical approach to sexual matters, which is concerned to understand sexual anomalies, and if necessary to treat them, but not to condemn them.

(Ellis, 1933, p.3 and pp.126–7)

Extract 4.2 Freud: 'The sexual life of human beings'

One would certainly have supposed that there could be no doubt as to what is to be understood by 'sexual'. First and foremost, what is sexual is something improper, something one ought not to talk about.

... it is not easy to decide what is covered by the concept 'sexual'. Perhaps the only suitable definition would be 'everything that is related to the distinction between the two sexes'. But you will regard that as colourless and too comprehensive. If you take the fact of the sexual act as the central point, you will perhaps define as sexual everything which, with a view to obtaining pleasure, is concerned with the body, and in particular with the sexual organs, of someone of the opposite sex, and which in the last resort aims at union of the genitals and the performance of the sexual act. But if so you will not be very far from the equation of what is sexual with what is improper ... If, on the other hand, you take the reproductive function as the nucleus of sexuality, you risk excluding a whole number of things which are not aimed at reproduction but which are certainly sexual, such as masturbation and perhaps even kissing ...

On the whole, indeed, when we come to think of it, we are not quite at a loss in regard to what it is that people call sexual. Something which combines a reference to the contrast between the sexes, to the search for pleasure, to the reproductive function and to the characteristic of something that is improper and must be kept secret – some such combination will serve for all practical purposes in everyday life. But for science that is not enough. By means of careful investigations (only made possible, indeed, by disinterested self-discipline) we have come to know groups of individuals whose 'sexual life' deviates in the most striking way from the usual picture of the average. Some of these 'perverse' people have, we might say, struck the distinction between the sexes off their programme. Only members of their own sex can rouse their sexual wishes; those of the other sex, and especially their sexual parts, are not a sexual object for them at all, and in extreme cases are an object of disgust. This implies, of course, that they have abandoned any share in reproduction. We call such people homosexuals or inverts. They are men and women who are often, though not always, irreproachably fashioned in other respects, of high intellectual and ethical development, the victims of this one fatal deviation. Through the mouth of their scientific spokesmen they represent themselves as a special variety of the human species – a 'third sex' which has the right to stand on an equal footing beside the other two.

(Freud, 1917, pp.344–6)

Extract 4.3 Kinsey et al., 'Sexual behaviour in the human male'

The six chief sources of orgasm for the human male are masturbation, nocturnal emissions, heterosexual petting, heterosexual intercourse, homosexual relations, and intercourse with animals of other species. The sum of the orgasms derived from these several sources constitutes the individual's total sexual outlet ...

There are some individuals who derive 100 per cent of their outlet from a single kind of sexual activity. Most persons regularly depend upon two or more sources of outlet; and there are some who may include all six of them in some short period of time. The mean number of outlets utilized by our more than 5000 males is between 2 and 3 ...

There are, both theoretically and in actuality, endless possibilities in combining these several sources of outlet and in the extent to which each of them contributes to the total picture … The record of a single sort of sexual activity, even though it be the one most frequently employed by a particular group of males, does not adequately portray the whole sexual life of that group … for marital intercourse may provide as little as 62 per cent of the orgasms of certain groups of married males … Again many persons who are rated 'homosexual' by their fellows in a school community, a prison population, or society at large, may be deriving only a small portion of their total outlet from that source. The fact that such a person may have had hundreds of heterosexual contacts will, in most cases, be completely ignored.

(Kinsey *et al.*, 1948, pp.193–4)

Extract 4.4 Hite, 'Sexual honesty'

[These are some responses of women to the questions: Is having sex important to you? What part does it play in your life?]

'Yes, having sex, which means being in love, is important to me. Having a good sexual relationship with my man is part of what our being together is all about.' (p.19)

'Not really. Lately I notice that I would just as soon not have it as have it.' (p.36)

'I'm not sure if having sex is important to me. Sometimes it is and sometimes it isn't. Outwardly I act indifferent about sex when I'm around other people. Inside myself, I think it's more important to me than it should be. I cover up how I feel about myself inside so no one will know.' (p.53)

'Yes, it is important to me to have it, now that I discover I am a sexual human being – I am 50 years old and two weeks ago I realized I only turned on to women. Sex is part of my love for women.' (p.80)

'Yes – mainly because it was a means of communication with someone I loved. Now I realize it is good for me to relax, let go and unwind this way. It is not the most important thing in my life by a long shot – but I think it is part of a well-rounded, well-balanced healthy life, psychologically and physically.' (p.85)

'Yes. There are about three ways through which I find a total release, a total sense of why humans live, a total sense of myself as a whole human being. These times are when working hard on my job, when orgasming, and when totally involved with another person, or especially with a group of persons, in a productive way. Thus, my sexuality is one of the most important aspects of my life, but only inasmuch as it is taken in the context of these other aspects that are so important to me.' (p.110)

'Yes, but it is considerably controlled. I am 16, living at home and a lesbian. For me, sex is a beautiful experience and important in showing my love to my lady and feeling my *sexual* love I have to hide so often.' (p.122)

(Hite, 1974, *passim*)

COMMENT

These extracts were chosen because the authors construct sex and sexuality in very different ways. For example, Ellis saw sex as an all-pervading aspect of a person's nature, something made up of different 'impulses' developing towards a permanent final outcome. He stressed the existence of wide variations in sexual behaviour, all of which are natural, and which can all be normal, so long as in some way they are

natural/
unnatural

associated with procreation. He saw abnormality in terms of 'deviations' from a norm which carry no moral judgements, but which may require treatment. He made clear that sexual attitudes and meanings have changed historically. Ellis was a sexologist (a scientist of sex) in the late nineteenth/early twentieth century, and he tried to adopt what he saw as the neutral value-free approach of a scientific expert. His view of sex as natural and biologically based was a challenge to earlier views of sexuality, which were framed in religious terms of sin.

Freud also saw himself as a scientific observer who could offer a detached view. He acknowledged the difficulties of defining 'sexual', which for him was about 'pleasure' associated with the body. From the end of the nineteenth century he developed the theory and practice of psychoanalysis, in which he emphasized the significance of unconscious sexual desires in human psychological development. He too acknowledged a wide variation among human beings, and identified particular kinds of people who differ from the average in terms of their 'object choice' (the object of their sexual desires). From this extract it is not easy to determine his attitude to these people.

In contrast, for Kinsey, a sexologist of the 1940s and 1950s, 'sex' was a particular kind of bodily activity that could be measured. A person's sexuality is defined in terms of all their possible 'sexual outlets', which for men can be achieved in six different ways. However, like Ellis and Freud, Kinsey stressed the diversity of human sexuality and as an 'expert' observer of 'facts', he was concerned to avoid judgements of 'normality' and 'abnormality'.

Shere Hite also saw herself as a sexologist, but used a very different methodology for obtaining information about sexuality. The women who filled in her questionnaire in the 1970s were not 'experts'; they were describing their own personal experiences and feelings, their sense of themselves, their subjectivity. What is most striking is the huge variations in the meanings they gave to sexuality: sex as a release of energy; as a way of relaxing and being healthy; as love or a means of communication; as a (lesbian) identity; and as something to be kept hidden – for one respondent even from herself.

■ ■ ■

2.3   Normality and deviance

There are both similarities and differences in the ways that sexuality is socially constructed in these accounts. To a large extent, for all the writers, people are defined by their sexuality. Whether focusing on people's nature, behaviour, feelings or identity, their sexuality tells us and themselves who they are. Sexuality is seen as an *essential characteristic* of the individual. They all acknowledge the existence of diversity, but for Ellis and Freud in particular, this is in a context

**normal/
abnormal**

of clear notions of normality and abnormality

What does 'normal' mean to you in the context of sexuality?

Common-sense views define 'normality' in terms of 'heterosexuality' as opposed to 'homosexuality' – what Freud described as a difference of 'sexual object choice', which is so significant that it creates distinct kinds of people (Extract 4.2). What is generally considered normal is those activities that are at least related to the possibility of procreation (Extract 4.1). As we saw in earlier chapters, one consequence of establishing a norm is that it is seen as unproblematic. Thus it is not considered necessary to explain heterosexuality, particularly heterosexuality that conforms to traditional moral principles of marriage and monogamy. Consequently, while there have been many studies into the causes of homosexuality, there have been very few studies of heterosexuality.

Indeed, attempts to study heterosexuality are very likely to meet with incredulity. When Kitzinger *et al.* invited 300 women who identified themselves as feminists to write 100 words on the contribution of their heterosexuality to their feminism, 'many many women wrote asking how they *knew* they were heterosexual, and, indeed, how *they* could tell whether they were heterosexual or not, and just what *is* a "heterosexual" anyway?' (Kitzinger *et al.*, 1992, p.297).

Most of the women who replied felt uncomfortable with the label 'heterosexual'. For example, one woman realized that it was an aspect of her identity that she had never previously considered. When she did, she recognized the privileges that such an identity carried for her:

> Of the many influences I have tried to find for my ideas and my work, my heterosexuality has not come to mind before … The status of heterosexual is a safe one and so has remained simply latent.

> Being heterosexual has several benefits. The first is that it means being 'ordinary'. Having said 'heterosexual', there is nothing to hide on that front. One's experiences can be shared with many others. There is one less reason for the children to be ashamed of one. One can enter into most cultural narratives, that is novels, films, fine art, on the basis of simple and satisfying identification.

> The second benefit, which I value as highly as the first, is that, with the required skill and energy, and a significant degree of luck, one can enter into and maintain the status of wife and of mother and have as a base for all of one's life, a family home. Others can have that, but the cement seems harder when a nexus has formal recognition all around.

> (Beloff, 1992, p.424)

Another woman had previously written about herself as heterosexual, but realized how different it was to be 'named' by someone else:

> That invitation produced in me the profound sense of being labelled. This had a salutary effect; through experiencing how the act of self-naming is radically different from the act of naming *the other*. To be invited to write *in the name of heterosexuality* by another is to experience the force of being positioned as Other. In this context, the name 'heterosexual' seems far more permanent and concrete than in my own use of it.

> (Young, 1992, p.423)

Assuming that heterosexuality is unproblematic suggests that heterosexuality and homosexuality are distinctive and exclusive forms of sexuality, and this is consistent with an essentialist approach to sexuality. One consequence of the focus on homosexuality in general is that lesbianism and male homosexuality are grouped together as different versions of the same deviation, and every individual is assumed to be *either* homosexual *or* heterosexual, with no space for 'bisexuality'. We shall return to these issues later.

But why is the distinction between heterosexuality and homosexuality seen as *the* crucial sexual difference between people? As we saw in Extract 4.4, people differ in many other ways: the importance that sexuality plays in their lives; the age of their first sexual relationship; how often they engage in sexual behaviour;

the kinds of behaviour they engage in; the number of partners they have; and the moral beliefs they hold. Even if these variations occur within heterosexual practices, the differences are not seen to be of equal value. Some sexual practices and some relationships are seen as morally 'better', more satisfying or naturally healthier than others. Consider, for example, the differential values placed on sexual intercourse within marriage compared with adultery, casual sexual encounters, sexual harassment or rape, or on 'same-race' compared with 'inter-racial' sexual relationships. The privileging of vaginal intercourse as 'real sex' means that in most countries legal definitions of rape must include vaginal penetration; that a woman who has engaged in a great deal of heterosexual sexual activity, but has not experienced penetration, would still technically be a virgin; and that lesbians cannot have 'real sex', only foreplay.

2.4 Diversity, difference and power: the creation of subject positions and identities

We saw in earlier chapters that different constructions are more than different words; they have important consequences for how people see themselves and are seen by others, as well for social intervention. We want to explore some of these consequences here. We shall start by considering the impact of a range of social differences on constructions of sexuality.

ACTIVITY 4.3

Read Extracts 4.5–4.11 and consider how particular groups of people are seen in relation to their sexuality.

1   What important dimensions of difference can you identify?

2   What views of natural and normal sexuality are expressed?

3   What normative standards of behaviour are prescribed?

Extract 4.5 Wilson: 'On human nature'

In most species, assertiveness is the most profitable male strategy. During the full period of time it takes to bring a fetus to term … one male can fertilize many females but a female can be fertilized by only one male … It pays males to be aggressive, hasty, fickle, and undiscriminating. In theory it is more profitable for females to be coy, to hold back until they can identify males with the best genes. In species that rear young, it is also important for the females to select males who are more likely to stay with them after insemination.

Human beings obey this biological principle faithfully. It is true that the thousands of existing societies are enormously variable in the details of their sexual mores and the division of labor between the sexes. This variation is based on culture … Nevertheless, this flexibility is not endless, and beneath it all lie general features that conform closely to the expectations from evolutionary theory …

We are, first of all, moderately polygynous, with males initiating most of the changes in sexual partnership … In diverse cultures men pursue and acquire, while women are protected and bartered. Sons sow wild oats and daughters risk being ruined. When sex is sold, men are usually the buyers.

(Wilson, 1978, pp.125–6)

Extract 4.6 Cowie and Lees: 'Slags or drags'

[The following quotes are taken from group discussions with teenage girls.]

'At least the girls we go with ain't second-hand.' (Conversation between boys baiting another boy – overheard by two girls in our study)

'When there's boys talking and you've been out with more than two, you're known as the crisp that they're passing round … The boy's alright but the girl's a bit of scum.' (Fifteen year old girl)

(Cowie and Lees, 1981, p.19)

Extract 4.7 *The Guardian*: 'Women's power "a turn-off" '

The empowerment of women over the past 10 years could be to blame for an increase in cases of impotence among men, according to a new report.

An analysis of 3,693 cases by the relationship counselling service, Relate, shows that almost a quarter of men receiving psychosexual therapy are now being treated for impotence. For the first time the disorder has replaced premature ejaculation as the most common sexual problem for which men seek help.

Counsellors say one reason for the increase is that men feel stripped of their masculinity as the power of women has increased in the workplace and in the bedroom.

According to a Relate counsellor, Julia Cole, some men fight back by saying they are not interested in sex, while others feel so emasculated that they are unable to perform.

(*The Guardian*, 16 April 1996, p.6)

Extract 4.8 Dollard: 'Caste and class in a southern town'

If Negro women are represented as sexually desirable in the folk imagination of the whites, Negro men are viewed as especially virile and capable in this sphere. The idea seems to be that they are more like savages, nearer to animals, and that their sexual appetites are more vigorous and ungoverned. There is a widespread belief that the genitalia of Negro males are larger than those of whites; this was repeatedly stated by white informants … It was further said that this impression was confirmed at the time of the draft examination of Negroes at the Southerntown Courthouse in 1917. Two physicians from other states have verified this report on the basis of draft-board experience. A Negro professional, on the other hand, did not believe that Negroes have larger genitalia than whites. He had worked in military camps where he had a chance to see recruits of both races naked, and said there is the usual variation within the races, but no uniform difference as between races …

It might not be worth the time of an actual research to determine the facts. One thing seems certain – that the actual differences between Negro and white genitalia cannot be as great as they seem to the whites; it is a question of the psychological size being greater than any actual differences could be. The belief is further suspect because the same point seems to be coming up with respect to the Jews in Germany, i.e., that they are at a competitive advantage in this respect and that sex relations with a non-Jewish woman are likely to be traumatic. This idea about genital size in Negroes is not mentioned because it is a curious belief or for the sake of noting a quaint exaggeration; the notion is heavily functional in reference to the supposed dangers of sexual contact of Negroes with white women.

(Dollard, 1949, pp.160–1)

Extract 4.9 Frankenberg: 'White women, race matters'

[Interviews with white women in California.]

'One white friend of mine introduced her boyfriend to me and he was Black, and I was just kind of shocked. In [my home town], that just would not be done … I know this sounds really racist. It *is* really racist. In high school you're taught anyway really strictly what is OK to do and what not to do around sex. And what we got really strongly is for a woman to have sex with a Black man is like being the worst slut in the world. I mean it's bad to be a slut anyway, but with a Black man it's so degrading.'

(Frankenberg, 1993, p.87)

Extract 4.10 Marshall: 'From sexual denigration to self-respect'

[Interviews with black women.]

'I think that many of the sexual images are sensual images. Black women are seen as sensually appealing. Often there's this dark mystical woman. Often Black women's figures, their shapes, are very different to 'white' women and so they're much more ample both above and below. I think that's seen as very sensual. I often think it's seen as off-limits. It's seen as if it's hot; it's too hot to handle.' (Tracy, p.12)

'It is 'white' men who see the Black woman as an unsatisfied mamma just to be used sexually … Black women are seen as sexual animals. For example, in the media they are beasts. The Black woman is an unsatiated mamma who can satisfy you. You are just to be used any way and not to be seen as a person. As a human being you are used and thrown away like rubbish.' (Sally, p.13)

(Marshall, 1996, pp.12–13)

Extract 4.11 Smith: 'Spinal cord injury'

I thought I knew all the facts – a man's sex was in his penis; if a man was a *man* he tried to 'score' whether he was interested or not. If he got a 'no', he still persisted. Other guys would talk about their conquests or their experiences. Most guys exchanged their information about sexuality in competitive environments like the locker room. They would say, 'I did this and that', and I would nod my head like I knew what was going on; to admit that I *didn't* know what was going on was to admit that I wasn't a man.

Then I broke my back body surfing in 1968 …

I felt asexual for a long time because a man's sex was supposed to be in his penis, and I couldn't feel my penis. So that contributed to my feelings of being asexual; it didn't occur to me that it felt good to have the back of my neck licked, or that it felt good to have my arms stroked lightly … I'm presently living with a man … I feel that we have a very equal relationship; I don't feel like I have to be the initiator all of the time.

(Smith, 1981, pp.12, 16)

It would seem from these extracts that people's sexual 'natures' are constructed in terms of a range of social differences. These differences are not equally valued, but are always defined in relation to a norm. In particular situations, any of the aspects of difference may be visible or focused on, so that what is defined as dominant or subordinate will vary, depending upon the particular norm that is operating. A power hierarchy is set up in terms of people who conform to the norm – whose sexuality is assumed to be unproblematic – and 'others' who are defined as problems in terms of their deviation from the norm.

■ ■ ■

Let us explore these examples further. Women and men are expected to be fundamentally different sexually, and their gendered natures vary in turn with 'race' and disablement. For Wilson, a sociobiologist (Extract 4.5), there are natural differences between women's and men's sexuality that derive from evolution. Men are naturally the initiators, fickle and undiscriminating, in contrast to women who are naturally coy and in need of protection. Extract 4.7 suggests that in 1996 women's sexuality expressed assertively was seen as pathological (unnatural) and hence dangerous to men, for whom 'sex' is about competition and conquest (Extract 4.11). A double standard of morality based on gender, evident in Extract 4.6, constructs two distinct classes of women, the 'Madonna' and the 'whore'. Extract 4.10 shows that these constructions are also racialized.

Although all men are assumed to have uncontrollable urges which women must both satisfy and keep under control, black men are 'more like savages, and nearer to animals', with voracious sexual appetites reflected in their assumed anatomical features (Extract 4.8). Note that, writing in the 1940s, Dollard uses the trem 'Negro', which was later rejected and replaced by 'coloured' and then 'Black'. Dollard uses the parallel with Jews in Germany to reinforce his argument that this is not based on 'facts', but is a construction which legitimizes ideas of black men as highly dangerous to white women, and of sexual relationships which cross 'racial' boundaries as unnatural, degrading and unacceptable. It also reflects anxieties and fantasies, which Freud attributed to men, about penis size and fear of castration, and about the sexual prowess of 'other' men. These assumptions about black men were shared by the white woman growing up in California in the 1970s (Extract 4.9). Frankenberg (1993) argues that underpinning these views is the idea of 'racial' differences as biological differences (recall Chapter 3). She suggests, from her interviews with white women, that by voluntarily engaging in such relationships, white women signal either inadequacy or perversion.

Assumptions about the gendered and racialized nature of sexuality automatically place black women within the category of deviant or sexual other, since they are seen to have a 'natural' pathological sexuality which is not only active but also either animalistic or exotic. Black women and men are constructed as homogeneous groups and as 'other'. Despite this homogenization, different groups of black women and men are also represented differently. The constructions we have been considering are applied in particular to women and men of African-American and Afro-Caribbean origin and descent. In contrast, advertisements for airlines and tourism, for example, regularly portray women from the Indian sub-continent and South East Asia as docile and exotic, and available to (white) men.

racialization

other

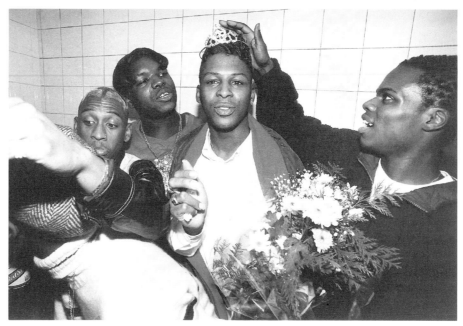

The winner of the Mr Black/Asian Gay and Bisexual Londoner Contest: a representation of gay liberation or a further representation of black male sexual prowess?

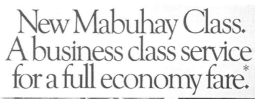

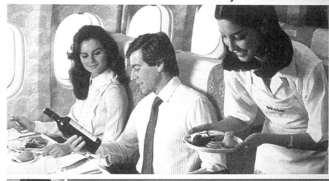

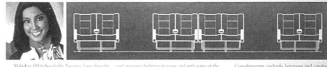

A racialized and gendered construction of sexuality

One important theme of this book is that such gendered and racialized discourses have important consequences. Constructions of women's sexuality can be understood in relation to reproduction and the family, so that how women are seen in terms of their sexuality has consequences for their capacity to be seen as 'proper' women and hence mothers, or as 'fit' mothers. So although the norms of acceptable femininity, linked to 'race', have changed historically, at all times women who deviate from the norm are likely to be seen as unable or unfit to be mothers. For instance, before 1873, adultery barred women from custody of their children, and in the 1870s Annie Besant lost custody of hers after publishing an 'obscene work' (an inexpensive pamphlet on birth control). More recently women who work as prostitutes and lesbian women have been seen by definition as incapable of being mothers, or have lost custody of their children purely on the grounds of their sexuality.

Racialized constructions of sexuality can be understood in terms of legacies of slavery and imperialism. Nineteenth-century Europeans thought that 'Africans had deviant sexual practices and searched for physiological differences, such as enlarged penises and malformed female genitalia, as indications of this deviant sexuality' (Collins, 1990, p.168). We can see how discourses are institutionalized in social arrangements and power: the exploitation, sexual violation and rape of black women has been justified by their portrayal as sex objects available for (white) men, as 'breeders', and as animals. Such discourses continue to produce, and be reproduced by, racist institutions and practices.

Similarly, the imperial relationship of domination and subordination between so-called 'Western' and 'oriental' societies is produced and reproduced in discourses of 'orientalism' which have constructed 'the East' (an area stretching from the eastern Mediterranean to Japan) as exotic, erotic, strange, passive, irrational and lazy, in contrast to 'Europe' as rational, virtuous, energetic, mature, normal and sexually ascetic. Within these discourses 'oriental' women and men are respectively sensual and inviting, effeminate and weak (Said, 1978; Turner, 1994).

Another context for understanding constructions of sexuality stems from fears in nineteenth-century Britain about the decline of the 'national stock', and concerns about the quality of the imperial 'race':

> The injunctions of nineteenth-century imperial propagandists to the young innocent – to be a 'man' and eschew masturbation, homosexuality or nameless other secret sins, or to embody motherhood and purity for the sake of the race – brought together class, race, gender and sexuality into a potent brew which locked normality and sexuality into a fixed hierarchy that few could escape from even if not so many lived up to it.
>
> (Weeks, 1995, p.87)

Summary

In the discussion so far we have suggested that 'sexuality' is socially constructed in different and contradictory ways – as behaviour, desires, practices, kinds of people. It is seen as a product of nature, and yet also influenced by social factors, and as something which involves moral choices. It is viewed as a fundamental characteristic of an individual that develops through childhood and adolescence towards the normative 'outcome' of heterosexuality. Norms of sexuality are both gendered and racialized, placing women and men within a hierarchical order according to different 'racial' characteristics. We have seen that these norms are also constructed in terms of disablement and age. You may wish to think about ways in which they are constructed through other factors such as class and nationality.

One of the important consequences of these different constructions is that they create our personal subjectivities, our sense of who we are, the choices and relationships we feel are available to us, and our social identities and positions in the world. In Extract 4.4 a woman described her feeling that sex was more important for her than it *should be* and felt she had to hide this from others. In Extract 4.11 a man who could not feel his penis or orchestrate a sexual encounter felt that he could not be a real man and must be asexual. The images of black women and men seem to define them entirely in terms of their bodies and their sexualities, and dehumanize them. We shall see later the importance of these issues, not only in placing people in the social world and for social intervention, but also for giving them a way of acting and organizing around those positions.

3   Essentialism versus social constructionism

3.1   Sexuality as an essential characteristic of people

A common feature of many of the accounts we have considered is that sexuality derives from 'natural' biological bodily processes. This approach originated in the work of the nineteenth-century sexologists, who, in their classification of varieties of human sexual practice, constructed sexuality as a powerful biological urge, an instinct (like hunger) which must be satisfied. Social influences on sexuality are acknowledged, but these are assumed to act on a biological base.

essentialism
hegemonic

This approach to sexuality is described as essentialism. Essentialist views of sexuality are hegemonic: they seem to fit with 'common sense', and appear to explain our subjective feelings by giving them a clear and unavoidable cause. In this book we have been arguing that such essentialist views are not statements of fact, but are social constructions.

Two features of essentialist ideas of sexuality are important for us here: first, sexuality is seen as natural, permanent and unchanging for individuals; second, apparently similar forms of behaviour occurring in different cultures or at different historical times are assumed to have the same personal and social meanings. What does vary historically and cross-culturally, according to this approach, is attitudes towards sexuality, and tolerance of particular aspects of sexual diversity. The last 150 years are seen in terms of a steady lifting of sexual repression and therefore movement towards greater tolerance and permissiveness.

Although essentialism is characterized by the features we have described, there are different versions of it. In particular, it has been linked with very different political agendas. In all cases 'natural sexuality' is seen as important for maintaining social relationships, and ultimately social order. For conservative thinkers natural sexuality is seen as uncontrolled and uncivilized: the basic biological force is potentially anti-social and destructive, and needs to be contained and controlled in the interests of a stable society. Unnatural forms are therefore 'deviant' and represent threats to the social order and are the sign of a decline of civilization. They should be 'stamped out', or at least tightly controlled. The 'traditional family', the stabilizing location for natural sexuality, is the cornerstone of society and should be supported. Young people are seen as particularly vulnerable to corruption and contagion, and therefore in need of protection.

In contrast, in the left-wing, libertarian version of this discourse, popular with radical groups in the so-called 'permissive 1960s', sex was seen as a powerful natural force which had been repressed and restricted within the confines of the nuclear family, in the interests of capitalism and patriarchy. 'Sexual liberation' was seen as a necessary part of the process of changing society and overthrowing capitalism. In most interpretations, however, heterosexuality was still seen as normal, with 'unnatural' forms being seen as a product of capitalist decadence.

There are also feminist versions of essentialism which argue that there is an inherent female sexuality that is common to all women and fundamentally different from men's, and that women should be encouraged to discover and satisfy their 'real needs' which have been repressed and distorted by patriarchy (see, for example, Sherfey, 1972).

3.2 Social constructionism: the challenge to essentialism

Within essentialist perspectives, cross-cultural and historical variations are understood as products of different or changed attitudes towards natural sexuality, and similar behaviours occurring in different circumstances are assumed to be examples of the same natural forms of sexuality. However, consideration of these same cross-cultural and historical variations contributed to challenges to essentialism and the development in the 1970s and beyond of an alternative perspective – that of social constructionism. This alternative approach rejects the idea of sexuality as a fixed, biological natural force shaped by social influences. On the contrary, it suggests that the meanings given to sexuality vary with specific social and historical circumstances, and that it only has meaning within socio-historical contexts.

social constructionism

A forerunner to this approach was the recognition from anthropological studies of the enormous variation in sexual practices in very diverse societies, and in particular the widespread occurrence of same-sex sexual behaviour. In line with essentialism, this was all described as 'homosexual'. However, comparative data from 190 different societies, summarized by Ford and Beach (1952), had identified 'two broad types of accepted patterns: the institutionalized homosexual role and the liaison between men and boys who are otherwise heterosexual' (McIntosh, 1968, p.186). The latter is a pattern also associated with Ancient Greece.

In an important paper, McIntosh (1968) questioned whether these different patterns should be understood as expressions of the same natural biological drive within different social contexts, as they seemed to represent completely different social meanings. In the second pattern 'there may be much homosexual behaviour, but there are no "homosexuals"' (McIntosh, 1968, p.187).

McIntosh similarly raised questions about historical research which tended to look back in time for 'great men' who could be fitted into modern stereotypes of 'homosexuality'. This search for historical equivalents to contemporary practices and identities increased as gay and lesbian liberation movements developed in the 1970s. As people who saw themselves as homosexual became more visible and self-confident in their identities, they wanted to search for their hidden 'roots'. McIntosh questioned this approach to history on the grounds that it can impose meanings that may not be appropriate. She suggested that historical change should be understood not as shifting attitudes, but as changing social constructions. For example, she claimed, before the end of the seventeenth century, the conception of homosexuality as a condition characterizing some individuals, or of 'the homosexual' as a kind of person, did not exist. Subsequent work has suggested different historical periods at which 'the homosexual' first appeared in Western societies, but the details of these debates are not important for us. Our concern is to recognize how questioning cross-cultural and historical evidence shows that the idea of a 'homosexual' as a kind of person only exists in some societies and at some historical times; therefore it is only in these socio-historical circumstances that it is possible to be a homosexual subject. This constitutes a challenge to essentialist accounts of sexuality, and opens up the possibility of an alternative social constructionist perspective.

Challenges to essentialism have also come from feminists, who reject the 'double standard' of morality, the idea that women have 'true needs', and the definition of heterosexuality in terms of men's needs. They reject essentialist ideas which justify women's oppression on the grounds that what is natural cannot be changed. Instead, they have struggled to make possible conditions in which women can achieve 'sexual liberation' (Jackson and Scott, 1996).

Before developing the arguments further, it is important to recognize that social constructionist approaches to sexuality should be understood in a dual way:

- First, they challenge the hegemony of essentialist views of sexuality as natural, arguing that these ideas are social constructions.

- Second, they offer an alternative view of sexuality, suggesting that sexuality itself is socially constructed.

Thus social constructionist views do not replace 'incorrect' essentialist ideas with the 'truth'. We are arguing that social constructionist ideas, like the essentialist positions, are alternative competing social constructions.

In order to explore this approach further it is important to refer to the ideas of Foucault (discussed in Chapters 1 and 2), which have had a major influence on the development of social constructionist positions on sexuality (Foucault, 1981). Within the essentialist approach, the Victorian period had been seen as a time of great sexual repression. Foucault challenged what he called the 'repressive hypothesis', suggesting that the Victorian period was not characterized by silence, denial and repression, but by a 'discursive explosion', a time of enormous interest in sexuality in which a new language developed through attempts to describe and classify forms of behaviour. New 'sexualities' such as homosexuality, nymphomania and fetishism were named for the first time and thought of as exclusive characteristics of particular kinds of deviant people. Hence they produced new 'subjects' like 'the homosexual' and the 'hysterical woman'. Sexuality was therefore not controlled through prohibition but through processes of 'normalization'. Central among these were views of the essentially different sexual natures of women and men, and of the natural superiority of heterosexuality.

For Foucault, the history of sexuality is a history of the discourses on sexuality that have been deployed within Western culture in the service of hierarchical relations within society. The naming of these deviant forms of sexuality by the medical and psychiatric professions, and their discovery within so-called 'normal' families, justified the intervention of a range of medical, psychiatric, legal and welfare experts. 'At stake in late nineteenth century Europe was the health of the "family" and its role in securing the health of the "race" … The "repressive hypothesis" itself served to mask the actual workings of power, which established sexual difference and heterosexuality as "natural" ' (Martin, 1991, p.15). Foucault also argued that, since this time, 'sex' has been located as the 'truth of our being', an essential characteristic of our true selves.

For essentialists, the history of sexuality is one of a gradual lifting of repression since the Victorian era. In contrast, historians of sexuality such as Weeks, influenced by Foucault, explore 'a variety of forces that have shaped and constructed "modern sexuality" ' (Weeks, 1981, p.12). Weeks argues that, in Western industrialized societies in the past 200 years, 'sex' has come to be a much more central feature of human life, seen predominantly in terms of sexual differences between women and men, and the normal/abnormal dichotomy of hetero-/homosexuality:

> The core of the historical argument has been that we can understand sexuality only through understanding the cultural meanings and the power relations which construct it … This does not mean that biology is irrelevant, nor that the body has no role … To say that lesbian and gay identities have a history, have not always existed and may not always exist, does not mean they are not important. Nor should it be taken to imply that homosexual proclivities are not deeply rooted. That question is in any case irrelevant to the argument. The real question does not lie in whether homosexuality is inborn or learnt. It lies instead in the question: what are the meanings that this particular culture gives to homosexual behaviour, however it may be caused, and what are the effects of those meanings on the ways in which individuals organize their sexual lives. That is a historical question. It is also a question which is highly political: it forces us to analyse the power relations which determine why this set of meanings, rather than that, are hegemonic; and poses the further question of how those meanings can be changed.
>
> (Weeks, 1995, p.7)

We saw earlier that, within an essentialist approach, homosexuality and heterosexuality are seen as distinct and exclusive forms of sexuality. In contrast, a social constructionist approach might want to emphasize that heterosexuality and homosexuality are defined in opposition to one another. Dollimore (1986) adopts this latter approach and also makes links to the way in which sexual subjects are produced. He argues that homophobia (fear of homosexuality) is used to define the limits of acceptable masculinity, so that being normally heterosexual is inseparable from, and conditional upon, not being abnormal.

Some feminists have also utilized Foucault's approach to challenge the distinction, described in section 2.1, between biological 'sex' and socially constructed 'gender'. They suggest that women's experiences of their bodies, feelings and desires are not biologically determined, but constructed through discourses of the female body (Crowley and Himmelweit, 1992). Foucault had described how the medical discourses of the nineteenth century constructed women in terms of their reproductive potential. Women were seen as ruled by their wombs, creating the idea of hysteria (a term that derives from the Greek word *hystera* for womb), and also creating the condition of hysteria that many middle-class women experienced: 'As the "subjects" of this discourse, nineteenth century women became, in some cases, literally hysterical' (Crowley and Himmelweit, 1992, p.64). In the late twentieth century women rarely experience hysteria, but other gendered 'disorders' such as anorexia nervosa have been understood in terms of contemporary discourses of the female body (Bordo, 1988).

What are the central features of a social constructionist approach to sexuality?

Vance (1989) suggests that:

> At minimum, all social construction approaches adopt the view that physically identical sexual acts may have varying social significance and subjective meaning depending on how they are defined and understood in different cultures and historical periods. Because a sexual act does not carry with it a universal social meaning, it follows that the relationship between sexual acts and sexual identities is not a fixed one, and it is projected from the observer's time and place at great peril. Cultures provide widely different categories, schemata, and labels for framing sexual and affective experiences. The relationship of sexual act and identity to sexual community is equally variable and complex. These distinctions, then, between sexual acts, identities, and communities are widely employed by constructionist writers.
>
> (Vance, 1989, p.18)

However, Vance (1989, p.19) also suggests that 'the increasing popularity ... of the term "social construction" ... made it appear that social construction is a unitary and singular approach'. In contrast, she emphasizes that there is more than one social constructionist approach, differing in terms of the range of aspects of sexuality seen as constructed. For the most radical form of constructionist theory,

> sexual impulse itself is constructed by culture and history ... [while] more middle-ground constructionist theory ... implicitly accepts an inherent sexual impulse which is then constructed in terms of acts, identity, community, and object choice ... [It is] evident that constructionists may well have arguments with each other, as well as with essentialists.
>
> (Vance, 1989, p.19)

Summary

In this section we have explored essentialist approaches to sexuality, which emphasize its natural basis for individuals and for particular social groups. Sexuality is assumed to have normal and abnormal forms, which can be found in different societies and at different historical periods. Cross-cultural and historical variations are attributed to changing attitudes and social controls.

In contrast, we have seen that for social constructionists there is no pure essence of sexuality on which controls operate; instead, sexuality itself is produced through processes of regulation and control. Its social and personal meanings therefore vary with socio-historical circumstances, and we have seen the dangers of applying labels and categories to different historical periods or to different societies.

In this chapter we have referred to several historical tendencies which help us to understand the construction of modern sexuality:

■ Developments in the family and the position of women from the middle of the eighteenth century (see also **Hall, 1998; Mooney, 1998**).

■ Legacies of slavery and imperialism which have helped to create particular discourses of sexuality relating to racialized women and men.

■ In nineteenth-century Britain, the strong fear of the decline of the 'national stock', and concern about the quality of the imperial 'race'.

■ The emergence of new discourses on sexuality in the nineteenth century, within various legal, medical and religious practices, which produced new sexual subjects.

4 Social constructionist views of sexuality: introduction to the case studies

In the rest of this chapter we want to illustrate social constructionism as an approach by focusing on two specific forms of sexual behaviour in Western industrial society which are defined by dominant forces as unnatural, abnormal and immoral: prostitution and homosexuality. The choice of homosexuality may seem obvious, as we have argued that in Western society the heterosexuality/ homosexuality dichotomy has been central in the construction of sexuality. Prostitution is included in order to demonstrate that this approach can also be applied to forms of heterosexual practice. We shall also see some interesting links and contrasts between the two examples.

These 'case studies' are therefore designed to demonstrate ways in which particular kinds of sexuality are created, and the effects of these constructions. In order to illustrate the importance of the social and historical context, and to show continuities and changes, we shall look in very general terms at three historical moments that have been important in shaping current views and discourses. These are: the late nineteenth century, the post Second World War period of the 1950s, and the late twentieth century from the 1970s on. As in Chapter 2's discussion of disability, we shall see how professional discourses, in this case legal and medical, became the expert knowledge on sexuality, and how these have been challenged.

4.1 The late nineteenth century

As a broad generalization, it is agreed that during the nineteenth century 'sexuality' was seen as a dangerous, corrupting and contagious force, which had to be contained and controlled by laws and policies which reinforced the middle-class family as the proper site for acceptable sexual activity. In the process, particular groups of people such as 'prostitutes' and 'homosexuals' were constructed as distinct from the norm. Dominant concerns about sexuality shifted from religious discourses of 'sin' to moral ones of 'vice' in the context of social concern about the health and purity of the 'nation'. Towards the end of the century, scientific studies of 'sexology', such as those of Havelock Ellis, were charting the existence of sexuality 'in nature', classifying and categorizing its different forms, challenging ideas of what was or wasn't 'natural', though retaining strong views on 'normality'.

4.2   The 1950s

In the period of the developing welfare state after the Second World War, in contrast to 'sex as danger', a fulfilling sexual relationship was viewed as an important source of social stability and personal happiness within the traditional family, the cornerstone of society. With an acceptance of the desirability of successful heterosexual sexuality within monogamous marriage, there was also a clear view of the importance of distinguishing between 'private' and 'public' behaviour and morals. Law and social policy were not seen as legitimate forms of intervention into the 'private' sphere of the normal family, but were there predominantly to control public nuisance. Particular social reforms in the 1960s (divorce, abortion, prostitution and homosexuality) were framed within this context, and have contributed to the social construction of this decade as one of 'sexual permissiveness'.

4.3   The 1970s

In the context of apparently greater freedoms, social movements developed, in particular feminism and gay liberation, which explicitly challenged dominant discourses of traditional morality and constructed new discourses of sexual liberation. Feminist debates emphasized 'choice' in sexuality represented by the demand of the Women's Liberation Movement for women to be able to define their own sexuality. The new discourses opened up possibilities for new subject positions, so that gay men and lesbians rejected ideas that they were sick or deviant and declared themselves 'glad to be gay'.

5   The social construction of prostitution

5.1   Contested definitions: what is prostitution?

In section 3.2 we suggested that what Foucault called the 'discursive explosion' on sexuality in the late nineteenth century helped to construct new kinds of people, including a particular class of women named as prostitutes. Prostitution itself was not new; on the contrary, what has often been described as the 'oldest profession' has been known at all times in history and in almost all societies. However, the social constructionist approach emphasizes that the use of the term 'prostitution' does not imply the same social meanings at different times and in different places. In turn, variations in social meanings alert us to the possibility of many different and contested definitions of prostitution.

How you would define 'prostitution'? Compare your ideas with the following dictionary definition:

'Of women: the offering of the body to indiscriminate lewdness for hire'

(*Shorter Oxford English Dictionary*, 1986, p.1691)

COMMENT

Reflecting on the dictionary definition, the following points occurred to me:

- It is traditionally assumed that prostitutes are women, but men can also be prostitutes, though generally with other men.
- Prostitution can involve heterosexual or homosexual sex.
- Women very rarely purchase sex.
- Prostitution is condemned as immoral (words like 'lewdness', 'base', 'abandoned' and 'corrupt' are used in further parts of the dictionary definition).

■ ■ ■

The dictionary reference to indiscriminate sexual activities in exchange for cash is open to many different interpretations. Perkins and Bennett comment that such a definition

> would not include, for instance, someone who has sexual intercourse with many people without accepting any money in return. Nor would it encompass people who marry purely for their partner's money … But it may be interpreted to include the woman who agrees to go to bed with men who dine her in a grand enough style … The very word 'indiscriminate' here may not be useful in describing a mistress granting sexual favours to the one man so long as he keeps giving her cash, handing her gifts and paying her rent, but can it be used to refer to the call-girl with only a half dozen regular clients? And is this call-girl very different from the career woman who has granted sexual favours to a number of men able to advance her position in the company? The call-girl and career woman … are probably closer in behaviour than either would be to the street prostitute. Do we then have to measure degrees of indiscrimination?

> If a person accepts cash once only for granting sexual favours it may be incorrect to assume that he or she is a prostitute; many feminists argue, on the other side, that a wife prostitutes by having sex with her husband in return for material comforts and financial security.

(Perkins and Bennett, 1985, pp.3–4)

Common-sense definitions imply that 'prostitutes' are distinct kinds of people. Alternatively, prostitution can be seen as a kind of occupation, or as a 'business transaction understood as such by the parties involved and in the nature of a short-term contract in which one or more people pay an agreed price to one or more other people for helping them attain sexual gratification by various methods' (Perkins and Bennett, 1985, p.4).

In this book we have emphasized that 'words matter', and we can illustrate this by considering the use and avoidance of the term 'prostitution' in particular situations. First, 'prostitution' groups together activities occurring in very different contexts: in the street, brothels or massage parlours, via escort agencies or through telephone advertisements in phone boxes. Those who view prostitution as an occupation are more likely to refer to 'sex work' or 'commercial sex', terms which also avoid the connotations of immorality. The 1990s saw a public recognition of the global dimensions of prostitution when what became known as 'sexual tourism' hit the headlines, a term which hides the particular power relations embedded in these practices.

> Sexual tourism promises jaded business men 'exotic' women in exotic locations, and should once more alert us to the intersections between gender, 'race' and class. Third World women are constructed as exotically other, as docile and hospitable waiting to welcome the traveller. This imagery pervades much of the marketing of regular tourism in South East Asia, and is easily transferred to commercial sex – the more so since it mirrors the wider market relationship between rich and poor nations. In the local context where young women are recruited, poverty is a major motivating factor for entry into sex work.
>
> (Jackson and Scott, 1996, p.25)

We see again here the racializing discourses on sexuality that were discussed in section 2.4. In another example, discourses on prostitution render invisible the exploitation of children. In the mid 1990s particular concern focused on the availability of children as prostitutes, both as part of sexual tourism and within the UK. The dominant view was that adult men paying for sexual activities with women as young as 12 or 13 years old was a form of prostitution, resulting often in prosecutions of the young women. This was contested by welfare workers and campaigners, who described such events as child abuse on the grounds that since young women under the age of 16 cannot consent legally to sexual intercourse, they cannot be prostitutes. Indeed, the campaigners demanded that the men be prosecuted and the children protected, but they have had great difficulty in getting their position recognized (Swann, 1997).

5.2   Essentialism: the inevitability of prostitution

Dominant ideas on prostitution are linked to the gendered and racialized social constructions of sexuality which we discussed in section 2.4. Although seen as morally reprehensible and a 'social evil', prostitution is nevertheless seen as universal and inevitable. This idea derives from the essentialist views of male and female sexuality discussed earlier in this chapter – the view that men 'need' sexual outlets and that women should satisfy these. However, as McIntosh (1978, p.54) says, 'Innately, it seems, women have sexual attractiveness while men have sexual urges ... No one worries about the needs of women'. Moreover, since men are responding to natural urges, while the women are going against their nature, the double standard of morality means that 'women are stigmatised as bad or fallen if they have casual sex or promiscuous sex', but 'casual, promiscuous or commercial sex is not seen as something conflicting with male sexuality; it is only when they turn to other men rather than to women that they are stigmatised' (Perkins and Bennett, 1985, p.13)

Prostitution has also been seen as providing a useful sexual service within society, for those men who for reasons of their social situation or personal characteristics cannot obtain sexual satisfaction in 'normal' ways: 'Enabling a small number of women to take care of the needs of a large number of men, it is the most convenient sexual outlet for an army, and for the legions of strangers, perverts, and physically repulsive in our midst' (Davis, 1937, p.755). In Chapter 2 we saw that disabled people are widely assumed to be sexually dysfunctional, and prostitution has sometimes been seen as a solution, but only for disabled men.

It also follows that women are not seen as the purchasers of sex. Working-class women, and women constructed as 'other' because of their 'race', are more likely than middle-class women to be seen as less respectable, immoral and more willing to engage in such degrading activities. We saw earlier the global dimensions of this. Later we shall see that racialized groups of men, both black and white, have often been positioned as the pimps, the real 'villains' who exploit prostitutes and make money out of the needs of otherwise respectable men.

Through these dominant discourses of sexuality, men's engagement with prostitution is naturalized and even justified, whilst its condemnation as an immoral activity is focused mainly on the women involved. Consequently, legislation and other forms of social intervention have been concerned to regulate prostitution rather than to suppress it, and it is the visible forms, particularly female street prostitution, that are seen to create a 'public nuisance' that must be controlled.

5.3   Historical changes and continuities: the late nineteenth century

By the 1850s prostitution had come to be seen as the 'great social evil'. It had symbolic importance, representing the worst aspects of social and moral degradation and thus the decline of the nation and the British (white) 'race'. The majority of the working class were seen as sexually depraved, constituting a threat to the moral and political order; prostitution was regarded as 'a source of pollution and a constant temptation to middle class sons' (Walkowitz, 1980, p.34). Literature in the mid Victorian period was pervaded by images of 'fallen women', the innocent victims of seduction and betrayal by middle- and upper-class men, and of children entrapped into prostitution. However, they were rarely distinguished from prostitutes, who were seen as depraved, brutal and a disgrace to their sex. Prostitution was not understood in terms of a woman's own social and cultural world. Yet full-time prostitutes in Victorian Britain often had an independent lifestyle and participated in a distinctive female subculture. Although poverty was a principal cause, the women were rarely starving: 'difficult circumstances precipitated the move into prostitution, [but] for many, that move still constituted a choice among a series of unpleasant alternatives' (Walkowitz, 1980, p.19).

The first attempts by the state to control prostitution occurred as part of wider concerns and intervention on public health. In the 1860s a series of Contagious Diseases Acts were passed in an attempt to control the spread of venereal disease among enlisted men in garrison towns, assumed to be spread by prostitutes. Under this legislation women identified as 'common prostitutes' were subjected to fortnightly internal examinations and, if found to be suffering from venereal disease, they could be interned for up to nine months in hospital. The definition of a 'common prostitute' was very vague, and it was up to the accused woman to prove her virtue. However, the Acts were never likely to be very successful in controlling disease as they applied only to women and not to men; indeed, there were violent objections to attempts to extend them to men.

An awkward encounter in Regent Street, London, 1871: 'That girl seems to know you, George!'

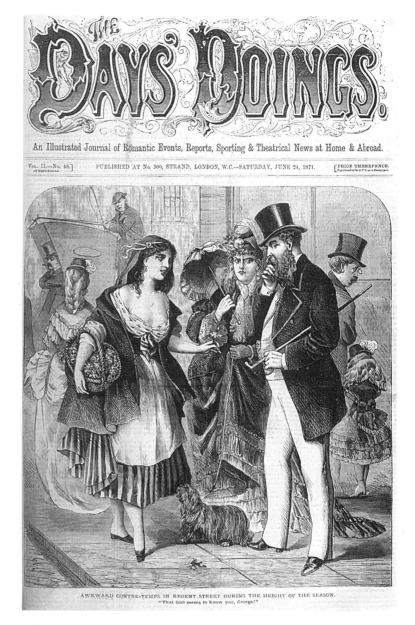

AWKWARD CONTRE-TEMPS IN REGENT STREET DURING THE HEIGHT OF THE SEASON.
"That Girl seems to know you, George!"

The Acts took for granted the double standard of sexual morality and accepted without question the existence of prostitution. The impossibility of distinguishing clearly between 'respectable' and 'fallen' women meant that all working-class women were kept under surveillance and constantly under suspicion of 'immorality', particularly if they appeared to be 'loitering' in the streets, an unnatural activity for women. Their 'respectability' and 'guilt' could be judged by their dress and appearance:

> They may be continually seen in their rooms pursuing their ordinary work without shoes or stockings, and with only a single garment on, secured by a petticoat tied around their hips … and in the same state they even continually walk through the streets in the middle of the day.
>
> (*London City Mission Magazine*, 1847, quoted in Barret-Ducrocq, 1991, p.11)

The surveillance of working-class women that took place under the Contagious Diseases Acts can be seen as part of the wider development of state intervention into the lives of the 'unrespectable poor'. Images of the poor were suffused with filth and contagion; they were seen as the 'great unwashed'. Thus 'literally and figuratively the prostitute was the conduit of infection to respectable society' (Walkowitz, 1980, p.4). Through the control of sexuality, the Contagious Diseases Acts could reinforce existing patterns of gender and class domination, as well as the divide between public and private life (**Hall, 1998; Mooney, 1998**).

Public opposition to these Acts developed strongly from the 1870s, resulting in their repeal in 1886. The opposition came from several quarters, and demonstrates both contested definitions of the 'social problem' and the consequences of these for different agendas for intervention. Middle-class nonconformist feminists stressed the importance of women's purity, moral supremacy and domestic virtue, and attacked what they saw as 'male sexual licence'. They therefore reinforced the ideology of separate male and female spheres. In contrast, within radical and socialist circles, critics of the Acts constructed the problem in terms of class and gender, focusing on and campaigning against the sexual exploitation of working-class women by middle-class men.

5.4 Prostitutes as types of women

Repeal of the Acts did not end the control of prostitutes, but it took new forms. The Criminal Law Amendment Act of 1885 attempted to suppress brothels, raised the age of consent to 16, and gave the police far greater jurisdiction over poor working-class women and girls (Walkowitz, 1980). These and later legislative measures helped to develop a much clearer boundary between acceptable and unacceptable women. Women working as prostitutes became socially isolated not in terms of what they did, but as distinct types of women.

Concern about the moral fabric and public health of the nation continued after the First World War, and women and girls spreading disease to men was again regarded as a prime cause. This is clearly reflected in the parliamentary debates on the Criminal Law Amendment Act 1921, which removed the defence of 'having reasonable cause to believe a girl was of, or above, the age of 16 years' from previous legislation on the age of consent.

ACTIVITY 4.5

Read Extract 4.12 from the parliamentary debate on this proposed amendment. How are prostitutes constructed in this extract?

Extract 4.12 *Hansard*: 'Parliamentary debate on the Criminal Law Amendment Act 1921'

[Major Farquharson, proposing the Bill, was concerned with 'the public health aspect':]

The very conditions in the last half century suggest to me that an enormous amount of physical disability which we found prevalent during the War in this country was directly traceable to the conditions of life during that past half century. I am perfectly certain that an enormous amount of the venereal disease which prevailed

– I would go so far as to say 80 per cent – was transmitted by children and very young persons.

… the attributes of a higher life and morality and religion are much more likely to be grounded upon a sure foundation given a clean, healthy body, than the reverse. I am perfectly convinced that the responsibilities of our race were never greater than at the present moment. Our domestic future, and in a great degree our international future, depends primarily upon the health of England. We won freedom in the 17th century. Britain had her triumphs of industrialism in the 18th and 19th century. If we desire to carry the civilisation, the industry, and commerce of the nation to the uttermost parts of the earth, we must not forget on the one hand one very vital thing … the soundness of the stock at home. England's breed, the culture of her race, the future destiny of this country depends to a great extent upon the culture of our race. This is a Bill for the protection of our race, and a stepping stone to a greater and a higher physical efficiency than we have secured in the past. (cols 1652–3)

[Major Lowther, opposing this clause:]

The age is fixed at 16. That is a very arbitrary age. It is not true that in all cases at 16 only does a girl reach the age of puberty … It is very largely a question of temperament and of nationality. There are in this country a large number of young aliens, especially, and I say it without offence, a large number of young Jewish women, Italians and Southerners who are plying the trade of prostitutes on the streets of London. They have the appearance of English girls of the age of 18 or 19, or even 20, and it is a very strong order to say that a man may not raise as a defence for having had intercourse with a girl of that kind that, although she was not yet 16, she was from appearance a girl of very much greater age. (cols 1661–2)

(*Hansard*, 15 July 1921)

COMMENT

Clear connections are being assumed here between sexuality, gender, 'race', nation and empire. The quality and health of the 'race' and 'nation', the future and greatness of England (sic) is seen to be threatened by 'young aliens'. This is an example of the racialization of a white group, as described in Chapter 3. These young women are seen as particularly dangerous because they look 'English', but have a very different nature; they are constructed as 'other' in terms of their temperament, nationality and bodily appearance.

■ ■ ■

5.5 The 1950s: contested definitions of public and private

Gender and 'race' continued to be important in constructions of prostitution during the post Second World War period of the 1950s. The liberalization of views of female sexuality meant that 'sex' was a key part of marital fulfilment for women as well as for men. But sex was still viewed as a 'duty' by women, and prostitutes were seen as 'folk devils', since they represented a threat to stable monogamous family relationships (Smart, 1981). Smart (p.49) suggests that the 1950s saw a 'successfully orchestrated moral panic' over prostitution, focused on two issues – tourism and the 'problem of immigration'. At the time of the Coronation there were large numbers of tourists in London, which was acquiring a 'shameful reputation … as the vice centre of the western world' (Smart, 1981, p.50). As in the 1920s, links were made between prostitution and 'race'; immorality and threats to the social order were linked to alien 'others' defined in terms of 'race' and nationality. In this period the racialization focused on the pimps and took a different form: 'In post war London many of the pimps were said to be Maltese, Italian and West Indian, and this combination of black or foreign men, said to be "living off the bodies of white women", was utilized to enrage public opinion' (Smart, 1981, p.50). Magistrates and judges spoke of a desire to bring back whipping, and MPs raised questions of deportation for black and foreign pimps. Note how the term 'foreign' is used to racialize groups of white men.

In 1954 the government had set up a Committee under Sir John Wolfenden to consider issues concerning homosexuality. Later, following public pressure, the problem of prostitution was added to its tasks. The guiding principle of the Committee's report was the distinction between law and morality, between public nuisance and private choices. Prostitution was seen as socially deplorable, but at the same time the Committee did not believe the law should be concerned with private morals.

We shall see later that the application of this public/private distinction to homosexuality led to limited but progressive reforms. However, the same principle applied to prostitution justified a severe increase in controls. Police powers were increased over those women who needed to be publicly visible to carry out their occupation as prostitutes. The 1959 Street Offences Act, which applied to England and Wales, made it an offence for a woman named as a 'common prostitute' to loiter or solicit in a street or public place for the purpose of prostitution. She became liable for arrest without a warrant. Note that prostitution itself remained legal, and that only a 'common prostitute' could be guilty of this offence. A woman was deemed a 'common prostitute' if she had been cautioned for soliciting on two previous occasions; once known in this way, she could be convicted on the basis of police evidence alone. Crucially, the prosecution did not have to show that anyone had been annoyed. Men could not be known as 'common prostitutes'. The Wolfenden Committee (1957) explicitly rejected the idea that there should be penalties for 'kerb crawling'.

Within a year of enactment of the law, police jurisdiction was extended, so that 'A woman who solicited from her doorway or window was deemed to be, for the purposes of the Act, *soliciting in the street*' (Smart, 1981, p.51). For this group of women 'privacy' therefore took on a very different meaning, and prostitutes continued to be constructed as people without the same rights as 'ordinary' or 'respectable' citizens. The impact of the legislation was precisely to increase the power and control of the pimps over whom there had supposedly been so much concern.

Unlike other areas of sexuality, there has been no liberalization of the law on prostitution since the 1959 Street Offences Act. The Criminal Justice Act 1982 did remove the penalty of imprisonment for soliciting or loitering, but women can be fined so severely that they cannot pay the fine and still end up in prison (Smart, 1995). There have been no government recommendations to remove the term 'common prostitute', nor to change the system of cautioning. In 1985 a private member's Bill for England and Wales was passed which retained existing laws relating to women, but added penalties for men who persistently solicit

public/private

Prostitution on the streets of London in the 1950s: the vice centre of the world?

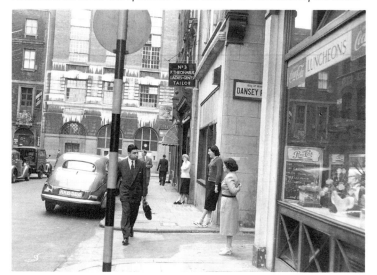
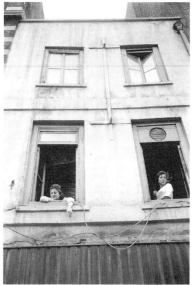

women for sexual purposes, and it made 'kerb crawling' an offence. Since the 1970s campaigning organizations have been established, largely by prostitutes themselves, to represent the interests of prostitutes and to campaign for the decriminalization of prostitution (see, for example, McLeod, 1982; Perkins and Bennett, 1985). In the late 1990s there were calls by some senior police officers to legalize brothels, and local authorities such as Edinburgh granted more licences to saunas and massage parlours, officially ignoring what takes place in them, in order to keep prostitutes off the streets. While supporters of these measures argued that this would be safer for the women, it nevertheless constituted a different form of control, leaving unaffected those who exploited the women involved.

5.6 Prostitution as a moral category

Why have views of the women involved in prostitution changed so little?

Smart (1995, p.55) suggests that, in line with common-sense ideas on female sexuality, 'most discussions of prostitution … invoke the cultural ideals of heterosexual love, monogamous marriage and the sanctity of the family'. In interviews with Sheffield magistrates in 1981, she found that marriage and the family were always the starting point for their views on the nature of prostitution. The magistrates all saw prostitutes as a 'distinct social category which was at some distance to "normal" or "respectable" people', and referred to them as '*these* people' or '*these* women' (Smart, 1995, p.60).

Smart argues that the law's ability to construct prostitutes as a special class reinforces common-sense views on prostitution which are in turn sustained by the legislation. She points out that modern laws on prostitution claim to be concerned with 'nuisance' rather than 'morality', but 'certain activities can only be legally defined as a nuisance if they are committed by a special, morally defined category of persons' (Smart, 1995, p.65). All the reports on prostitution since Wolfenden have:

justified the retention of a special law to regulate the nuisance caused by prostitution by reference to the fact that people find this kind of nuisance especially repugnant. What they fail to acknowledge is that 'nuisance' caused by a prostitute is more objectionable than 'nuisance' caused by a street vendor precisely because she is regarded as immoral. In other words 'nuisance' is just a moral category by another name.

(Smart, 1995, p.65)

Smart suggests that this 'logic' is based on attitudes towards prostitute women, which are so much part of 'common sense' as to be invisible. Such attitudes place prostitute women in a special class, whether as immoral or inadequate, to be disapproved of or pitied. These attitudes have consequences for all women, as they define the boundaries of decency and indecency.

ACTIVITY 4.6

In this section we have seen how social constructionism can help us to deconstruct dominant ideas on prostitution. Read the following extracts from parliamentary debates on (a) the Street Offences Bill 1959; (b) a private member's Bill introduced in 1979 by Labour MP Maureen Colquhoun to establish one single street offence; and (c) the Sexual Offences Act 1985.

1 What competing constructions of sexuality can you identify?

2 What are their implications for viewing prostitution?

3 What are the consequences for intervention?

4 In what ways are these constructions gendered and racialized?

5 What continuities and changes are there?

Extract 4.13 *Hansard*: 'Parliamentary debate on Street Offences Bill 1959'

[Mr Butler, Home Secretary, introducing the Bill:]

It is not the object of the Bill to make prostitution illegal, or to provide a cure for prostitution. The history of the world at any rate would show this to be impossible, at any rate by statute. The object of the Bill is to help clear the streets. (col. 1271)

I hope that the Bill will discourage women from adopting this way of life and remove some of the temptations to which young people are now exposed, I hope that we shall not only deal with conditions in the streets which constitute a public nuisance, but also make a positive and valuable contribution to the discouragement of vice and the redemption of those who are in danger of adopting it as a way of life. (col. 1275)

It will thus be asked why a single composite Clause cannot be inserted in the Bill dealing with men and women together. The fact is that men and women present different problems and cannot be dealt with in the same way … The women are easily identifiable; the men are not. (cols 1283–4)

[Lena Jeger opposed the Bill:]

It is quite clear from the Wolfenden Report, and from this Bill, that we do not know why girls take to the streets, or why men take to girls who take to the streets. Several hon. Members have referred to the disgrace caused by these girls being on our streets. No one has yet referred to the disgrace caused by men who pay these girls to stand in our streets … It is a discriminating measure by which an attempt is made to deal with the supply without dealing with the source of the demand. (col. 1319)

I find it an extraordinary reversal of our cherished ideal that we are all equal before the law. This Bill will create a section of the community, a section of third class citizens, to whom these principles do not apply. (col. 1320)

I should equally like to name some men as common frequenters of prostitutes. (col. 1324)

(*Hansard*, 29 January 1959)

Extract 4.14 *Hansard*: 'Parliamentary debate on Bill to establish one single street offence'

[Maureen Colqhoun, introducing the Bill:]

The Bill will establish one single offence to cover all persistent street nuisances, not only soliciting, and evidence from the person or persons annoyed will be an absolute requirement. The offence will include kerb-crawling, persistent salesmen, drunks and members of religious sects who attempt to sell people records on the street. I emphasise that it is only the peculiar sexual hypocrisy of the British that would single out prostitution as an offence. (cols 1094–5)

Finally, I emphasise that prostitutes and prostitution are not a menace. I have spoken with many eminent psychiatrists who say that it is accepted in their profession that prostitutes have great therapeutic value in society … Many psychiatrists accept that prostitutes are the oldest therapists in the world and are practitioners of professional therapy. (cols 1095–6)

[The Reverend Ian Paisley, opposing the Bill:]

I do so because I believe in the sanctity of our womenfolk … the standards that have made this nation and protected its womenfolk in the past are in serious jeopardy. (col. 1096)

The person who has been caught up in prostitution through exploitation, victimisation or by her own choice, has lost the greatest thing in life – the purpose for which she came into the world. She has lost her goal. All of us here today remember our own mothers, and thank God for them. We all remember the sanctity of the family and the joy and peace which flows from family life … This is only the beginning of a scheme to undermine what lies at the very heart of the moral fabric of our society. (cols 1097–8)

(*Hansard*, 6 March 1979)

Extract 4.15 *Hansard*: 'Parliamentary debate on Sexual Offences Act 1985'

[In introducing the second reading of the Bill, Janet Fookes quoted from a woman who had written to her:]

'For years now I have been unable to walk out of my flat without being accosted by men in cars. They wink at me, flash their lights, ride alongside of me, speak to me and even offer to up the price … Irrespective of what I am wearing these men, both English and foreign and some of them obviously well-educated, see me as a street walker. I can be carrying shopping from Sainsburys, dirty washing to the launderette, riding my bicycle, walking the dog round the square … The time of day is of no consequence either. I can be dashing to Sainsburys at 5 pm on Saturday, going to work at 8.30 am and coming home at 6 pm. Need I say more?' (col. 1244)

[Tom Cox, supporting the Bill:]

Motorists are to be seen driving around for hour after hour looking for prostitutes … any woman who walks along the streets of some areas – areas which have been invaded by kerb crawlers – will be seen as a potential prostitute. They can be young schoolgirls or elderly ladies who are pensioners. They can be walking home from school or going home from work. I have even been contacted by women to tell me they have been stopped by motorists when taking their young children out. They have been seen as potential prostitutes. One can understand their disgust. (col. 1249)

Prostitution has existed for a long time. I am sure that none of us thinks that we will be able to stop it … If we want to rid our streets of kerb crawlers, we must also consider whether it is time for a change in the law to allow women to advertise their services as prostitutes. (col. 1251)

(*Hansard*, 25 January 1985)

COMMENT

In these extracts prostitution is widely seen as inevitable, but different conclusions are drawn from this. Butler wished to control its public nuisance aspects, and to discourage young people from this 'vice', whereas Cox used inevitability as an argument for seeing prostitution in a different way, as a service that can be openly advertised, and thereby stopping the harassment of 'innocent' women.

You may have noted that concern about the gender discrimination within the law, present in the opposition to the 1959 Bill, was a central component of the 1979 and 1985 Bills. Colqhoun's proposals, which failed to become law, are particularly interesting. She challenged the construction of 'prostitutes' as a distinct class of women, and 'prostitution' as a special class of public nuisance. At the same time she accepts without question the dominant discourses of male and female sexuality, which see men as having 'sexual needs', when she describes prostitutes as the 'oldest' therapists in the world.

The extracts from the 1985 debate focus explicitly upon the nuisance caused by men who solicit women, but nevertheless strongly reinforce the construction of 'prostitutes' as 'other', as a category of women distinct from 'ordinary' or 'respectable' women. For an ordinary woman to be considered a prostitute was deemed quite horrific, and the horror was extreme if the ordinary woman was young, elderly or a mother. Motherhood and prostitution were clearly incompatible. The men who frequent prostitutes were also 'othered', but in this case in terms of 'class' and 'race', since the horror seemed to reside in the idea that they may be English and well-educated. The idea of uncontrollable male sexuality is reinforced by the observation that these men seek prostitutes at all times of the day or night.

■ ■ ■

Summary

This section of the chapter has explored competing constructions of prostitution, showing their historical specificity. We have seen the power of legal discourses and practices to construct women working as prostitutes as a distinct category of women, different from all other women, and how this intersects with other social divisions so that it is working-class and 'racially' subordinated women who are most likely to be categorized in this way. Exploration of the concern to regulate public nuisance has demonstrated varying social meanings of 'public' and 'private' as well as the importance of morality in defining a particular set of activities as a nuisance.

6　The social construction of homosexuality

Let us now turn to our second illustration by examining social constructionism in relation to homosexuality.

6.1　Contested definitions

ACTIVITY 4.7

Note down some possible ways of defining homosexuality. It may be helpful to skim back through the chapter to remind yourself of points already raised.

COMMENT

The definition of homosexuality, like that of prostitution, is not straightforward. It is possible to think about homosexuality in many different ways, for example as:

- same-sex sexual practices
- a sexual identity
- a gender identity (homosexual men and women are not seen as 'properly' masculine or feminine)
- patterns of non-sexual behaviour (for example cross dressing)
- a 'third sex' (see Extract 4.2)
- close same-sex emotional friendships (this is more commonly applied to lesbians)
- a medical condition
- an innate (genetically determined) predisposition
- an immoral choice.

However homosexuality is constructed, it is nearly always considered abnormal.

■　■　■

In section 3.2 we saw that many of the challenges to essentialist views of sexuality developed out of considerations of homosexuality, in particular the recognition that different social meanings may be attached to same-sex sexual practices occurring in a wide range of societies and at different historical times. We also saw that the idea of 'the homosexual' as a distinct kind of person or fixed identity, as opposed to ideas about 'homosexual acts', has emerged historically, and that homosexuality and heterosexuality are defined in opposition to one another. As a consequence, although male and female sexuality are constructed quite differently, male and female homosexuality are seen as similar forms of deviance:

they are both defined as essentially sexual and as 'not heterosexual'. The meanings given to homosexuality and lesbianism vary enormously, and they are fiercely contested even among those who identify themselves as homosexual or lesbian. (Plummer, 1992, p.14) states that homosexuality is not a 'unitary phenomenon … What we have are a multiplicity of feelings, genders, behaviours, identities, relationships, locales, religions, work experiences, reproductive capacities, child-rearing practices, political disagreements, and so forth, that have been appropriated by a few rough categories like "homosexual", "lesbian", "gay".'

6.2 Legal and medical discourses construct homosexuality

The law has played a crucial role in constructing 'homosexuality'. From 1885 to 1967, all homosexual acts between men, whether in public or in private, were illegal. Prior to 1885 the only relevant legal control was of 'acts of sodomy', which were seen as sinful and 'equally condemned as being "against nature", whether between man and woman, man and beast, or man and man' (Weeks, 1977, p.12). Crucially, the law attempted to control 'acts' or 'behaviour'; it contained no notions of 'homosexuals' as distinct kinds of people. The term 'buggery' was used to describe any activities not related to reproduction, from 'sodomy' to 'birth control'.

A crucial development was the passing in 1885 of the Labouchère Amendment to the Criminal Law Amendment Act. For the first time all male homosexual acts were criminalized, whether in public or private, and whether or not they involved sodomy. The law was strengthened still further in 1889 with the Vagrancy Act, which aimed to stop homosexual soliciting. Both Acts were primarily concerned with the control of prostitution, but for the Victorian 'social purity' campaigns, male homosexuality and prostitution were both symptoms of 'national decline', and products of men's uncontrollable lust. The impact of the new laws was most visible in a series of famous sensational trials, in particular those which led to the imprisonment of Oscar Wilde in 1895.

At the same time as these legal developments, medical 'experts' on sexuality were offering scientific accounts of the variety of sexual behaviour to be found among human beings. Rather than drawing a rigid line between procreative and non-procreative sex, the sexologists were classifying and distinguishing between many different forms of non-procreative sex, described variously as 'perversions' and 'deviations'. We saw in Chapter 2 the rise to dominance of a medical model of disability as an example of an 'expert' discourse which comes to 'own' a problem. Similarly, by the end of the nineteenth century, medical discourses of homosexuality were beginning to replace those of 'sin' or 'vice'. Homosexuality, now a distinct category, was seen as a naturally occurring form of sexuality, though still an aberration of nature and hence abnormal. It was further subdivided into its congenital and acquired forms. Congenital homosexuals or 'inverts' were also sometimes seen as a 'third' or 'intermediate' sex (look again at Extract 4.2). This construction allowed writers to call for more liberal responses to homosexuality, arguing the pointlessness of criminalizing something that was 'natural'. The shift in emphasis from moral to medical discourses, though morality has never disappeared, gave power to doctors and the search for causes and cures for homosexuality. Medical discourses caught on gradually but were incorporated into common-sense perceptions of homosexuality up to the 1960s, where they dominated the debates on reform (Weeks, 1977).

It is important to realize how the medical and legal discourses helped to construct, for the first time, new 'subjects' called 'homosexuals'; these discourses also had particular consequences for intervention. The sexologists had opened up possibilities for sexual experience and behaviour by challenging the taken-for-granted distinctions between natural and unnatural sexualities. However, at the same time they rigidified those possibilities by creating fixed categories into which people could be fitted, which restricted choice and made it easier to regulate or control them. As with prostitution, the law helped to draw a clear dividing line between acceptable and unacceptable forms of behaviour, placing homosexuals on the 'wrong' side of the law. However, according to Weeks (1977, p.21), 'in attempting to suppress homosexuality completely, our society actually gives rise to a greater incidence of exclusively homosexual individuals than other societies which make some provision in their mores for homosexual tendencies'. The humiliation of Oscar Wilde, says Weeks (p.21), 'helped to give a name to his predilection'. On the one hand, these new laws had a devastating effect on the lives of those individuals who could be prosecuted for their behaviour, and who feared such public disgrace. On the other hand, the very process of categorization also made resistance possible. People defined by the discourse as 'homosexuals' could identify themselves within it, and develop solidarity with others of the same group.

6.3   The construction of 'private life': the 1950s and 1960s – the era of reform

At a time of social stability and economic boom, with a renewed emphasis on family life, the dominant view of homosexuality was derived from medical discourses: the law was seen to blight the lives of individuals, who suffered from 'arrested development' and who were to be pitied.

In any case, the law was largely ineffective. Campaigns to change the law existed in Europe and the USA, and it seemed possible that the emphasis on a right to one's private life, free of state intervention, which for most 'normal' people would be found within the family, could be extended to homosexuals. Changes in public opinion and attitudes within the church, together with pressure from reforming groups, led to the setting up of the Wolfenden Committee to consider the law and practice relating to homosexual offences and the way people convicted of such offences were treated by the courts. We saw in section 5.5 that this same Committee was later asked to look at the law in relation to prostitution, and thus 'lashed together, in nineteenth century fashion, homosexuality and prostitution [although] its conclusion, by applying a single pragmatic criterion, finally separated them, both emotionally and legislatively' (Weeks, 1977, p.165).

The Wolfenden Committee recommended in its 1957 report that homosexual behaviour between two adult men over 21, in private, should be removed from the control of the criminal law. However, the Committee thought that the law should continue its dual role of protecting young people (defined as those under 21) and of preserving public order and decency. They therefore recommended that homosexual behaviour between adult males in public should continue to be a criminal offence.

Despite several attempts at reform, it was not until 1967 that legislation along these lines was enacted, and then it only applied to England and Wales. While constituting an important progressive reform, it was also very limited in scope, because of the age restriction of 21 (in comparison with an age of consent for heterosexuality of 16), and because of the narrow definition of 'private'. For example, a room in a hotel was legally a 'public' place.

ACTIVITY 4.8

Read Extract 4.16, which is taken from the parliamentary debates on a private member's Bill, introduced in 1966 by the Labour MP Leo Abse, on reforming the law on male homosexuality. Note down the dominant discourses on homosexuality. How are they linked to the forms of intervention proposed?

Extract 4.16 *Hansard*: 'Parliamentary debate on the Sexual Offences (No.2) Bill 1966'

[Leo Abse, introducing his private member's Bill on 5 July 1966:]

No one suggests that the House approves of fornication, adultery or lesbianism because we do not catalogue them in a list of crimes. Nor would any such approval be extended to homosexual activities by the Bill, particularly as, in so many instances, homosexual conduct would remain a crime attracting the most severe penalties. But the Bill would mean that the burden of criminality would no longer be attached to acts committed in private between adults. (col. 260)

Can the law be said to be a deterrent? How would we married men respond to a law enforcing celibacy upon us? Would we be deterred? Since these wretched men have similar compulsions, only, lamentably, directed to men and not women, how is it credible that the law acts as a deterrent? (cols 260–1)

[The law] prevents the integration of hundreds of thousands of our fellow citizens into the community, for any person who suffers the appalling misfortune of being a homosexual is bound to be under the gravest burdens … they are permanently denied the blessings of family life, the gifts and rewards of parenthood, the gift of a mature love with a woman. (col. 261)

Yet I believe that the worst failure of the present law is the preoccupation with punishment of homosexuals which leads to the community not taking the preventative action which might possibly save a little boy from the terrible fate of growing up a homosexual. Little as we know of the etiology, certain it is that there are dangers to a boy if an over-possessive mother ties him to her with a silver cord, so that the boy, enveloped in a feminine aura, is never able to break out and assert his masculine independence.

Equally certain it is that among fatherless boys there is a disturbingly high rate of homosexuals. A lad without a father, lacking a male figure with whom to identify, is sometimes left with a curse, for such it must be, of a male body encasing a feminine soul. If such are some of the precipitating causes of the ambiguity of the sexual rule amongst these people, who, with any compassion, can demand that to one disability in childhood must be added the stigma of criminality in adulthood?

All in this House … wish to see a diminution in the incidence of homosexuality. But I believe that education in mothercraft and, what is perhaps even more important, education in fathercraft, the mobilising of our social resources to lend more aid to the fatherless, the provision of more male child care officers and more male teachers are far more likely to succeed in this respect than praying in aid our penal system. (col. 262)

[Captain Elliot, in opposing the Bill on its second reading on 19 December 1966:]

I think it is worth considering the side effects of the Bill. We should, I presume, get a succession of plays on television and on the stage on the subject. We should get more books on it. We should get more clubs. I believe that the vice would be looked upon as a normal and natural part of our daily life, and all checks would be gone.

I sincerely believe that if the Bill is passed it will increase homosexual practices and not reduce them. It will not cleanse the national bloodstream; it will corrupt and poison it. It will not bring more happiness; it will bring greater misery. (col. 1082)

(*Hansard*, 5 July and 19 December 1966)

COMMENT

It is clear that Abse, whilst in favour of reform, was nevertheless at pains to express his disapproval of homosexuality, and to assert the need for severe penalties for its 'public' manifestations. He viewed homosexuality as a misfortune rather than a vice, something that could be explained in terms of abnormal psychological development. He saw it as a compulsion, similar in strength to that of normal male heterosexuality. Intervention to reduce the incidence of homosexuality was posed in terms of education for mothercraft and fathercraft. The argument for changing the law was therefore based not on any challenge to the view that homosexuality was abnormal, but firmly on the Wolfenden principle of the inappropriateness of the criminal law in relation to private behaviour among adults.

On the other hand, the reform was opposed on nineteenth-century grounds of the unnaturalness of homosexuality, and of the threat it posed to the very fabric of society, through the corruption and poisoning of the 'national bloodstream'.

■ ■ ■

6.4   Lesbianism – the importance of gender

In contrast to male homosexuality, lesbianism has never been criminalized, although it has been subject to social regulation. The nineteenth-century sexologists had found it difficult to find much evidence for female homosexuality. Where there was evidence, it was frequently linked to prostitution. This does not mean that women did not have relationships with other women, which may or may not have included sexual aspects, but there was no language in which to understand these as 'homosexuality' (Faderman, 1981). Havelock Ellis saw women who did display an active sexuality, independently of men, as 'true inverts' and particularly masculine.

In 1921 an attempt was made to criminalize lesbianism by adding a clause to the 1885 Criminal Law Amendment Act. This clause, passed by the House of

Commons, was rejected by the House of Lords, who persuaded the Commons of its controversial nature, the difficulty of gaining evidence, and the increased potential for blackmail. Supporters of the clause described lesbianism as a 'moral weakness', a 'beastly subject', and an 'objectionable vice'. In line with views on male homosexuality discussed earlier, there was a fear that if not controlled it would become the

> beginning of the nation's downfall. The falling away of feminine morality was to a large extent the cause of the destruction of the early Grecian civilization, and still more the cause of the downfall of the Roman Empire … this House … should consider it to be its duty to do its best to stamp out an evil which is capable of sapping the highest and the best in civilization.
>
> (Mr Macquisten MP, *Hansard*, 4 August 1921, cols 1799–1800)

However, opposition to criminalization was constructed in terms distinctive to lesbianism. Equally horrified by lesbianism, the opponents of the clause were concerned that it would have the unfortunate consequences of increasing the very behaviour it intended to stamp out. Colonel Wedgwood assumed that very few 'decent' people had even heard of lesbianism, and that 'it is being better advertised by the moving of this Clause than in any other way' (*Hansard*, 4 August 1921, col. 1800).

Lt Col. Moore Brabazon feared that if the clause were passed, it 'would do harm by introducing into the minds of perfectly innocent people the most revolting thoughts' (col. 1806). Similarly in the House of Lords, the Earl of Desart was 'strongly of the opinion that the mere discussion of subjects of this sort tends, in the minds of unbalanced people, of whom there are many, to create the idea of an offence of which the enormous majority of them have never even heard' (*Hansard*, 15 August 1921, col. 572). He was concerned that if there were any prosecutions,

> the results would be even more appalling. It would be made public to thousands of people that there was this offence; that there was such a horror. It would be widely read … I am sure that a prosecution would really be a very great public danger. Is there any necessity for it? How many people does one suppose really are so vile, so unbalanced, so neurotic, so decadent as to do this? You may say there are a number of them, but it would be, at most, an extremely small minority, and you are going to tell the whole world that there is such an offence, to bring it to the notice of women who have never heard of it, never thought of it, never dreamed of it.
>
> (*Hansard*, 15 August 1921, col. 573)

We can see that the debate about lesbianism was shaped by the nineteenth-century discourses of moral degeneracy and fears of national decline. The lack of any criminal laws or public sensations had meant that there was little if any public debate or knowledge of lesbianism. In the context of silence and lack of knowledge, it was difficult for women to construct for themselves any sort of lesbian identity. The MPs who opposed the proposed clause feared, perhaps rightly, that even to talk about it publicly would create the knowledge that would enable the identities to be formed.

An important public event in the 1920s did help to construct a lesbian identity. In 1928, Radclyffe Hall, an established prize-winning novelist, published *The Well of Loneliness*. In this novel, Hall set out to tell the 'truth' about lesbianism. She utilized Ellis's essentialist model of congenital inversion, arguing that if lesbianism is inborn it should be tolerated by society. Shortly after its publication, an introduction to the book by Ellis was the subject of a scathing attack in the

Sunday Express, calling for the book to be banned under the 1857 Obscene Publications Act. The attack focused on the presentation of lesbianism as innate, rather than as a decadent immoral choice. Ruehl (1982) suggests that the argument was essentially over definitions of lesbianism. The book, not the author, was on trial, so it was the publishers who were found guilty of obscenity and the book was banned. Ruehl's explanation for the verdict is that 'the concept of *lesbianism* itself ... was seen as dangerous, because the idea of "congenital inversion" allowed inverts to be described as attractive personalities and especially because it freed them from moral blame ... What was being fought over in the court was not simply the description, but the redefinition of lesbianism' (Ruehl, 1982, p.30). Ruehl (p.27) sees Hall's contribution as 'the start of a "reverse discourse", a process by which a category of lesbianism derived from a medical discourse is firstly adopted and then transformed by those defined by it ... her intervention in itself was both an adoption of Ellis's category of "inversion" and an initial step towards transforming it.'

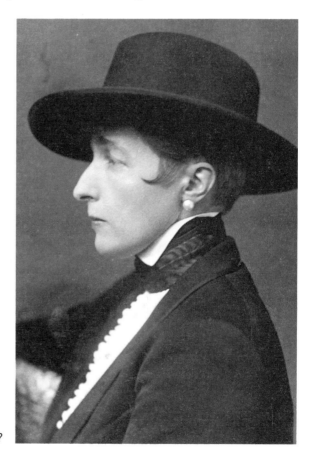

Radclyffe Hall in 1928: a particular definition of lesbianism?

The existence of female homosexuality would seem to challenge fundamental ideas on the 'nature' of women and their relationship to men. If women's sexuality is naturally passive to be awakened by men, how can lesbianism exist at all? Richardson (1992, p.191) suggests that the dominant 'phallocentric view of sex as penis in vagina meant sex between women was less easy to categorize as sexual and that therefore there was less pressure to restrict erotic interests in the same sex. It rendered sex between women as more invisible, but also more harmless.' This is illustrated in the 1966 parliamentary debate on male homosexuality, when the existence of lesbianism was acknowledged, but not seen to be in need of legal control since it did not create the same kind of social problems:

> The personality and nature of women are distinguishable from the personality and nature of men – because of the strength of their sexual initiatives and drives – and … the effect in society of lesbian women is not so potent as that of homosexual men. Nobody knows or hears of women being corrupted on a large scale by lesbian women, whereas I do not think that even the doughty champion of the Bill would deny that many male homosexuals are of the proselytising type.
>
> (Mr Iremonger MP, *Hansard*, 19 December 1966, cols 1104–5)

6.5   The construction of gay subjects

The 1967 reforms, like the events of the late nineteenth century, contributed to the development of new discourses around a new name for homosexuality and lesbianism – 'gay' – which created new possibilities for subject positions, group solidarity, resistance and social movements. It is important to recognize that 'gay' is not just a new label for 'homosexuality'; it constructs a new kind of person. In the same way that we cannot talk about 'homosexuals' before their construction as such in the late nineteenth century, we cannot look back in history and see 'gay' men and women. Rather than being seen as 'sinful', 'immoral', 'having a condition' or 'being arrested in their development', gay men and women since the 1970s have been able to assert their positive sense of self through slogans such as 'glad to be gay'. In a context of fewer legal constraints, a great emphasis was placed on the process of 'coming out', which had a dual function of acknowledging oneself as a gay man or lesbian, and declaring this publicly. The different gender experiences of women and men meant that 'gay' was still generally interpreted as male, while many homosexual women, particularly those involved with feminism, preferred to assert themselves as lesbians.

We have seen that social constructionism has been very influential in challenging the taken-for-granted common-sense views of homosexuality as a deviant aberration from normal heterosexuality. It opened up possibilities of developing a different history of homosexuality from the conventional one. Gay and lesbian writers have argued that this approach also allows space for differences in the constructions of lesbianism and male homosexuality, and for diversity among gay men and lesbians to be acknowledged. It also challenges the common-sense idea that it is only deviant sexualities like homosexuality that need to be studied and understood. For constructionist approaches all sexual roles and identities, including heterosexuality, can be studied in their socio-historical context (Fuss, 1989).

However, social constructionist approaches are open to different interpretations. For many gay and lesbian activists asserting for themselves a new non-pathological identity as 'gay', social constructionism appeared to deny the possibility of reclaiming a history and naming gay ancestors. In campaigning for further changes in the law, and an end to all forms of discrimination, activists achieved solidarity from asserting their 'essential nature' as lesbians and gay men. As a 'fixed minority' it was possible to demand, and begin to obtain, equality

subject
positions

181

with the heterosexual majority in all aspects of life, including those which recognized them not only as individuals but also within relationships. Lesbians also reasserted their identities as women, and many saw themselves as, and became, mothers, something the 'congenital inverts' of Radclyffe Hall's day were not able to do. At the same time they were positioned as 'lesbian mothers', and constructed as a social problem.

Britain a prime offender in EC on anti-gay laws

Gay couples given housing rights

California gays marry en masse

MPs vote to keep forces ban on gays

European court's gay sex ruling could embarrass Tories

More lesbian parents win

Runcie admits breaking ban on homosexual priests

The myth of the gay gene

MEPs back gay and lesbian right to marry

Newspaper headlines from the mid 1990s (Source: The Guardian, The Daily Telegraph, The Independent, The Observer)

For some lesbians and gay men, therefore, social constructionism is an approach that creates uncertainties. If history is about changing meanings, rather than about changing attitudes to a fixed 'essence', then presumably those meanings can change again. Weeks (1995) suggests that it feels safer to assert a permanent sense of self, rooted in nature. Thus some gay men have welcomed scientific claims of the discovery of a 'gay gene' (exclusively male so far).

In section 3.1 we argued that essentialism could not be associated with any particular set of values or political agenda. Similarly, social constructionism, though associated with sexual liberation movements, cannot be linked to any political values. New Right attempts to revitalize traditional morality in the 1980s saw 'deviant' lifestyles not as natural diversity, but as immoral choices which must be controlled in the interests of social order. The Local Government Act 1987–1988 included a controversial and much fought-over Section 28, which suggested that sexuality was not fixed, but could be 'promoted', and which sought to ban the 'promotion' of homosexuality in schools and in any situation involving local authority funding.

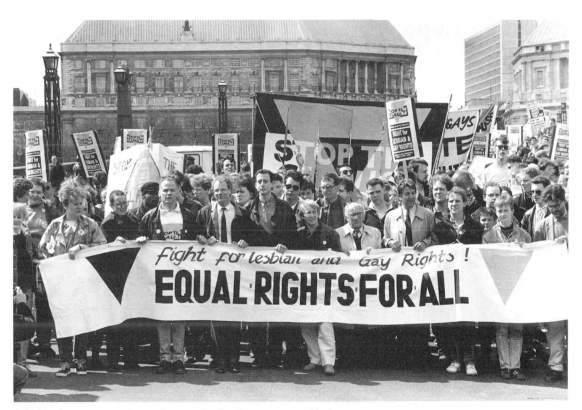

A 1980s demonstration demanding equal rights for gay men and lesbians

Despite greater freedoms and visibility, until 1994 male homosexual behaviour remained criminalized except between consenting adults over 21 in private. The laws in Scotland and Northern Ireland were brought into line with England and Wales in 1980 and 1982 respectively. In 1994 an attempt was made to reduce the age of consent to 16, in line with that for heterosexuality, through an amendment to the Criminal Justice and Public Order Bill. The outcome was a reduction in the age of consent from 21 to 18 in Britain, but not in Northern Ireland. At the time of writing (1997) this decision is being challenged in the European Court, as UK law is more restrictive than that of most other European Union countries.

ACTIVITY 4.9

Read Extract 4.17, which presents excerpts from the 1994 parliamentary debate on the lowering of the age of consent for homosexual acts. Try to identify continuities and change in comparison with the 1967 debate (look back at Activity 4.8).

Extract 4.17 *Hansard*: 'Parliamentary debate on amendment to Criminal Justice and Public Order Bill 1994'

[Edwina Currie, introducing the amendment on its first reading on 11 January 1994:]

We are talking about our fellow citizens. Gay men are people who we know, work with and like. What they do is not a disease and whether they do it or not is, and should be, entirely a private matter. I believe that the time has come to give those men the equality under the law which the rest of us take for granted. I believe that the choices they freely make are entitled to be treated with respect. (col. 69)

[Bill Walker, opposing the amendment on its second reading on 21 February 1994:]

Does the hon. Lady realize that it is neither natural nor normal to carry out homosexual activity? That is why there has to be protection for young boys. It is a different matter if they participate in that which is normal and natural, but if they are guided into activities that are neither normal nor natural, protection is required. (col. 79)

[Neil Kinnock, as a co-sponsor of the amendment:]

Let us tell young people that a heterosexual life, in the sense that it is what most of us live and want to live, is the norm; that it is and will remain the basic human relationship upon which the family is founded. But let us also tell young homosexuals that we still have regard for them and want them to live in a society that accepts their nature and will give them the same chance as others for personal happiness. We shall not tolerate discrimination against them and they need not feel fear and outlawed. Let us tell them that they can participate as fully as anyone else in the responsibilities and privileges of citizenship. (col. 86)

[Tony Blair, supporting the amendment:]

The overwhelming evidence – scientific or indeed merely experience of life – suggests that being homosexual is not something that people catch or are taught or persuaded into, but something that they are. It is not against the nature of gay people to be gay; it is in fact their nature. It is what they are; it is different, but that is not a ground for discrimination. (col. 98)

[The Reverend Ian Paisley, opposing the amendment:]

This country must realize that the unit of society, and the cement that holds it together, is the family. As goes the family, so will the nation. If we do not have the cement of the family, society will disintegrate and be destroyed … The normal sex act within the marriage vow, bringing together male and female and producing offspring, is the happy way; it is the divine way; it is the creative way; and it is the best way. As one of the apostles said, it is the more excellent way. (col. 114)

(*Hansard*, 11 January and 21 February 1994)

There were some very significant changes between 1967 and 1994 in the way that homosexuality was discussed. In 1994, the term 'homosexual' was used interchangeably with 'gay men', and being 'gay' or 'homosexual' was seen as part of one's 'nature' rather than as a medical condition or vice. The essentialist approach is seen most strongly in Blair's contribution to the debate. The argument for reform was no longer based on condemnation of homosexuality, but instead on the discriminatory aspect of the law in comparison with heterosexuality, denying equal citizenship to a particular class of young men. However, there are some continuities too. In Kinnock's speech, the norm of heterosexuality was strongly reinforced, and the element of pity for an unfortunate minority is still present. Gay men, he argued, should have equal rights, even though, through no fault of their own, they are unable to live up to the heterosexual ideal. Opposition to the amendment continued to be posed in terms of the threat to the nation, though in 1994 this was described in terms of weakening the 'cement' of the family, in contrast to the concerns in 1967 about the 'national bloodstream'.

7 Conclusion

In this chapter we have used an exploration of social constructionism in relation to sexuality to explore further many of the concepts and themes discussed in Chapter 1. As in Chapters 2 and 3, which focused on disability and 'race', we have seen the way in which definitions are contested and historically specific, and the role that social movements can play in this process of contestation.

This chapter has also demonstrated the power of normalizing discourses of heterosexuality to construct those who do not conform in one aspect of their behaviour or identity as particular kinds of people such as prostitutes, lesbians and homosexuals. It has also demonstrated their power to organize social intervention to deal with the resultant 'social problems'. At the same time the production of new subject positions has allowed groups of people to organize around those positions and to resist the dominant discourses. Our examination has shown also the importance of morality and the construction of the distinction between public and private life for regulating and controlling those excluded as abnormal or deviant. In addition, this process of 'othering' involves the intersection of sexuality with other social differences, particularly those of gender, class and 'race'.

We have also seen that social constructionism is itself not a unitary approach. In relation to sexuality, social constructionists disagree on the range of aspects of sexuality they see as socially constructed. It is also not an approach that can be associated with any particular social or political agenda.

As in Chapters 2 and 3, we have seen the solidity of social constructions and the significant and often devastating consequences they have for how we see ourselves, are seen by others, and for the choices we feel we can make. They also have material effects on people's lives. Women working as prostitutes, and lesbians and gay men are seen as a threat to the moral and social order, and we have seen that all these groups may be denied full citizenship simply on the basis of their sexuality.

Further reading

There are many places where you can read more on the debates between essentialist and social constructionist approaches to sexuality, for example Weeks (1981, 1985), Plummer (1992), and Jackson and Scott (1996). It is also helpful to look back at the important paper by McIntosh (1968), which is reproduced with a postscript in Plummer (1981); at Vance (1989), who offers a critical evaluation of social constructionist approaches; and at the very important and influential ideas of Foucault (1981).

One of the most prolific writers in the UK on sexuality from a social constructionist perspective is the historian Jeffrey Weeks; the development of his ideas can be followed in Weeks (1977, 1981, 1985, 1995 and 1996). He also explores, in the earlier works, the influence of the work of Freud and the sexologists on modern conceptions of sexuality.

The work of the sexologists Ellis and Kinsey is also discussed in Robinson (1976), while Freud's ideas can be found in the 1977 Penguin edition of Freud's collected writings on sexuality.

Feminist ideas and debates on sexuality since the 1970s are discussed in Jackson and Scott (1996). The essentialist/social constructionist debate and its implications for feminism are explored more fully in Spelman (1988) and Fuss (1989). A discussion of some of the issues around disablement and sexuality can be found in Bullard and Knight (1981).

For discussions of the boundaries and intersections between 'race', class, gender and sexuality, see Davis (1982), who focuses on the formation of gendered social relations in the USA, and Mercer and Julien (1988), who offer an analysis of the images and construction of black male sexuality.

Many of the references already given discuss issues of lesbianism and homosexuality. To read more on prostitution see Walkowitz (1980) for the nineteenth century, and Smart (1981, 1995) for an analysis of events in the 1950s and more recently. McLeod (1982) and Perkins and Bennett (1985) explore the experiences of women working as prostitutes and the development of their own campaigning organizations.

References

Barret-Ducrocq, F. (1991) *Love in the Time of Victoria,* London, Verso.

Beloff, H. (1992) 'On being ordinary', *Feminism and Psychology,* vol.2, no.3, pp.424–6.

Bordo, S. (1988) 'Anorexia nervosa: psychopathology as the crystallization of culture', in Diamond, I. and Quinby, L. (eds) *Feminism and Foucault: Reflections on Resistance,* Boston MA, North Eastern University Press.

Bullard, D.G. and Knight, S.E. (eds) (1981) *Sexuality and Physical Disability,* London, The C.V. Mosby Company.

Collins, P. Hill (1990) *Black Feminist Thought,* New York, Routledge.

Cowie, C. and Lees, S. (1981) 'Slags or drags', *Feminist Review,* no.9, pp.17–31.

Crowley, H. and Himmelweit, S. (1992) *Knowing Women,* Cambridge, Polity Press.

Davis, A. (1982) *Women, Race and Class*, London, The Women's Press.

Davis, K. (1937) 'The sociology of prostitution', *American Sociological Review*, vol.2, pp.744–55.

Dollard, J. (1949) *Caste and Class in a Southern Town*, second edn, New York, Harper and Brothers.

Dollimore, J. (1986) 'Homophobia and sexual difference', *Oxford Literary Review*, vol.8, no.1–2, pp.5–12.

Ellis, H. (1933) *Psychology of Sex*, London, Whitefriars Press.

Faderman, L. (1981) *Surpassing the Love of Men: Romantic Friendship and Love between Women from the Renaissance to the Present*, London, Junctions.

Ford, C.S. and Beach, F.A. (1952) *Patterns of Sexual Behaviour*, London, Methuen.

Foucault, M. (1981) *The History of Sexuality, Volume 1*, Harmondsworth, Penguin.

Frankenberg, R. (1993) *White Women, Race Matters*, London, Routledge.

Freud, S. (1917) 'The sexual life of human beings', reprinted in Freud, S. (1973) *Introductory Lectures on Psychoanalysis*, Harmondsworth, Penguin.

Freud, S. (1905–31) Collected writings on sexuality, reprinted in Freud, S. (1977) *On Sexuality*, Harmondsworth, Penguin.

Fuss, D. (1989) *Essentially Speaking*, New York, Routledge.

Hall, M. R. (1928) *The Well of Loneliness*, reprinted 1981, London, Virago.

Hall, C. (1998) 'A family for nation and empire', in Lewis, G. (ed.) *Formimg Nation, Framing Welfare*, London, Routledge in association with The Open University.

Hite, S. (1974) *Sexual Honesty*, New York, Warner Books.

Jackson, S. and Scott, S. (1996) 'Sexual skirmishes and feminist factions: twenty-five years of debate on women and sexuality', in Jackson, S. and Scott, S. (eds) *Feminism and Sexuality*, Edinburgh, Edinburgh University Press.

Kinsey, A.C., Pomeroy, W.B. and Martin, C.E. (1948) *Sexual Behaviour in the Human Male*, London, W.B. Saunders.

Kitzinger, C., Wilkinson, S. and Perkins, R. (1992) 'Theorizing heterosexuality', *Feminism and Psychology*, vol.2, no.3, pp.293–324.

Marshall, A. (1996) 'From sexual denigration to self-respect', in Jarrett-Macauley, D. (ed.) *Reconstructing Womanhood, Reconstructing Feminism*, London, Routledge.

Martin, B. (1991) *Woman and Modernity,* London, Cornell University Press.

McIntosh, M. (1968) 'The homosexual role', *Social Problems*, vol.16, no.2, pp.182–92.

McIntosh, M. (1978) 'Who needs prostitutes?', in Smart, C. and Smart, B. (eds) *Women, Sexuality and Social Control*, London, Routledge and Kegan Paul.

McLeod, E. (1982) *Women Working: Prostitution Now*, London, Croom Helm.

Mercer, K. and Julien, I. (1988) 'Race, sexual politics and black masculinity: a dossier', in Chapman, R. and Rutherford, J. (eds) *Male Order: Unwrapping Masculinity*, London, Lawrence and Wishart.

Mooney, G. (1998) 'Remoralizing the poor? Gender, class and philanthropy in Victorian Britain', in Lewis, G. (ed.) *Forming Nation,*

Framing Welfare, London, Routledge in association with The Open University.

Perkins, R. and Bennett, G. (1985) *Being a Prostitute*, London, Allen and Unwin.

Plummer, K. (ed.) (1981) *The Making of the Modern Homosexual*, London, Hutchinson.

Plummer, K. (1992) 'Speaking its name: inventing a gay and lesbian studies', in Plummer, K. (ed.) *Modern Homosexualities*, London, Routledge.

Richardson, D. (1992) 'Constructing lesbian sexualities', in Plummer, K. (ed.) *Modern Homosexualities*, London, Routledge.

Robinson, P. (1976) *The Modernization of Sex*, New York, Harper and Row.

Ruehl, S. (1982) 'Inverts and experts: Radclyffe Hall and the lesbian identity', in Brunt, R. and Rowan, C. (eds) *Feminism, Culture and Politics*, London, Lawrence and Wishart.

Said, E. (1978) *Orientalism*, London, Routledge and Kegan Paul.

Sherfey, M.J. (1972) *The Nature and Evolution of Female Sexuality*, New York, Random House.

Smart, C. (1981) 'Law and the control of women's sexuality: the case of the 1950s', in Hutter, B. and Williams, G. (eds) *Controlling Women*, London, Croom Helm.

Smart, C. (1995) *Law, Crime and Sexuality*, London, Sage.

Smith, D. (1981) 'Spinal cord injury', in Bullard, D.G. and Knight, S.E. (eds) *Sexuality and Physical Disability*, London, The C.V. Mosby Company.

Spelman, E.V. (1988) *Inessential Woman: Problems of Exclusion in Feminist Thought*, Boston, Beacon Press.

Swann, S. (1997) 'Commercial sexual exploitation of children – an issue of "prostitution" or "protection"', in Hayman, S. (ed.) *Child Sexual Abuse: Myth and Reality*, London, Institute for the Study and Treatment of Delinquency.

Turner, B.S. (1994) *Orientalism, Post Modernism and Globalism*, London, Routledge.

Vance, C. (1989) 'Social construction theory: problems in the history of sexuality', in Altman, D. *et al.* (eds) *Homosexuality, Which Homosexuality?*, London, GMP Publishers.

Walkowitz, J. (1980) *Prostitution and Victorian Society*, Cambridge, Cambridge University Press.

Weeks, J. (1977) *Coming Out,* London, Quartet.

Weeks, J. (1981) *Sex, Politics and Society*, London, Longman.

Weeks, J. (1985) *Sexuality and its Discontents*, London, Routledge.

Weeks, J. (1995) *Invented Moralities*, Cambridge, Polity Press.

Weeks, J. (1996) 'The idea of a sexual community', *Soundings*, no.2, pp.71–84.

Wilson, E.O. (1978) *On Human Nature*, London, Harvard.

Wolfenden Committee (1957) *Report of the Committee on Homosexual Offences and Prostitution*, Cmnd 247, London, HMSO.

Young, A. (1992) 'The authority of the name', *Feminism and Psychology*, vol.2, no.3, pp.422–4.

CHAPTER 5

Review

by Esther Saraga

Contents

1   Introduction

This book has examined a particular way of looking at and analysing the social world in which we live. It has focused mainly on how differences between people are perceived and interpreted, and how they are constructed as social problems. It has also looked at the consequences of these constructions for social intervention, and for how people see themselves and are seen by others. Whether or not issues such as poverty, lone parenting, disability, 'race' and sexuality are important issues for you personally, they are frequently addressed in everyday conversations and jokes, in fiction, in the press, and on television and radio. We have stressed that *how* these issues are talked about is very dependent on the social and historical context; indeed, in some situations they may be 'taboo', to be avoided. The specific topics that have been addressed in this book are likely to be familiar to most readers, even if the way in which they have been discussed has involved new concepts and ideas.

Chapters 2, 3 and 4 considered three aspects of social differences – those linked to disability, 'race' and sexuality. We looked in these chapters at the way different 'types' of people are produced as what we have called 'subjects' – in this case, people who are seen as different from 'normal' people and as particular kinds of 'social problems', and about whom something must be done through legal, medical or social policy intervention.

In each chapter it was stressed that the specific topics examined were not the central focus. Rather they were vehicles for exploring *social constructionism*, a particular approach to social science which was outlined in Chapter 1. We could have chosen a wide variety of alternative topics instead. In Chapter 1 we used a range of examples, including poverty, motherhood, lone parenthood, unemployment and age, and we could have considered any of these in greater detail. We might have also discussed the social constructionist approach through an examination of the social differences of gender or class, by looking at the life stages of childhood, adolescence and old age, or we could have considered social problems like homelessness, crime, child abuse or drug abuse.

On the other hand, the choice of topics was not arbitrary. First, they were selected because they are all useful ways of exploring particular themes, namely:

- The way social differences are *naturalized*.

- The categorization of people into groups and their construction as distinct homogeneous types of people, or 'subjects'.

- The consequences of these constructions for how people see themselves and are seen by others, and for forms of social intervention.

Second, the complexity of the themes is highlighted by the contrasts provided by these aspects of difference. By reading across the whole book, we can see the different ways in which the themes are manifested in particular contexts, and the different consequences of this for particular groups in society.

Finally, disability, 'race' and sexuality are also important topics in their own right, and the analyses offered in each chapter, though necessarily selective, will be of great value in further studies of social welfare and social policy.

The aim of this review chapter is not simply to summarize each of the preceding chapters, but to:

- Re-examine the themes outlined in Chapter 1 in the light of the way they were explored and illustrated in the following three chapters on disability, 'race' and sexualities.

- Compare and contrast ideas from the three chapters in order to elaborate further the central themes of the book.

- Consider how the general approach to social science, introduced in this book, can be applied more widely to analysing processes of social differentiation, social problems, and their relationship to social policy.

2   The social constructionist approach

Primarily this book has been concerned to examine social constructionism as a particular approach within social science. In the different chapters it has become clear that there are different ways of discussing social constructionism. Chapter 1 suggested that what the different ways have in common is 'their stress on the way in which collective or shared understandings, interpretations or representations of the world shape our actions within it' (p.29). The subsequent chapters have explored further the way in which social constructionist approaches are concerned with social meanings which themselves are linked to the relations of power that predominate. They also considered how those meanings are embedded, or become 'solidified', in social institutions, policies and practices, which in turn empower people to act in particular ways and help to legitimate existing social arrangements. In addition, they offered a range of examples of how constructions produce types of people described as 'subjects'. Crucially they have demonstrated that social constructions are contested: the language used to define terms, the explanations for problems and their solutions are all sites of struggle in which power relations are acted out.

In developing the social constructionist approach the following themes were outlined in Chapter 1 and explored further in the subsequent chapters:

- common sense and social science
- the naturalization of the social
- social differences and social problems
- contestation and power
- the consequences of social constructions.

In the sections that follow we shall explore each of these themes in turn, selecting examples from individual chapters to illustrate particular points. This review chapter will not cover all the issues and examples in each chapter, and you may therefore wish to recall other examples.

3   Common sense and social science

A major theme of the book has been the way we all take for granted certain aspects of the world we inhabit. The majority of people do not question the idea that disabled people, black people, gay men, lesbians and prostitutes are 'different', and that they may constitute social problems, though there may be disagreements over whether these groups of people *have* problems or *are* problems, over what kinds of problems they are, and how the problems should be dealt with. Our own relationship to these issues is likely to have an effect on how we view them – we shall explore this further in section 3.1.

Everyone constantly makes assumptions about people and the nature of the social world. Usually we categorize them into types, and then assume that we know all sorts of things about them. This is how we go about our daily business of living, and mostly we are not aware of doing it. In the process of categorizing people, and ascribing meaning to those categories, we make implicit assumptions about normality, about the nature of the differences between people, about what issues constitute social problems, about the kinds of problems they are, and about how they should be solved.

This book has been emphasizing the need to be a sceptical stranger in this familiar world of ours, to make explicit these implicit assumptions, to question these 'common senses' that are taken for granted, and 'to scrutinize "what everybody knows", alongside public, political and policy definitions of the problem and to disentangle the constructions that we find' (Chapter 1, p.12). Whoever we are, however we understand or interpret these issues – whether we agree with the dominant sets of ideas, or wish to challenge them – we need to ask questions such as:

■   Who says so?

■   What interests do they represent?

■   Why do they say this? (What assumptions are they making?)

■   How do they justify their views?

■   What are the implications of their assumptions?

Why do we refer above to common senses, in the plural?

Chapters 2 and 4 both referred to common senses in the plural. We did this to emphasize that there is not just one common sense that is simple and straightforward. Chapter 1 showed that statements about 'what everybody knows' evoke widely divergent views. Common sense is itself divided and contested, representing a 'storeroom' of all the bits of knowledge people use when discussing issues and problems in society. Common sense was described in Chapter 1 as 'conflicting and contested social claims', each of which implies that everybody shares the assumptions that underlie it. Although there are many 'common senses', there is usually *one* that becomes *the* common sense; that is, it is the dominant or hegemonic one which is most widely accepted as 'truth'. Part of the concern of all the chapters in this book is to deconstruct common sense.

Before reading further, look back over the chapters in the book and note down some of the examples of 'common senses' that have been analysed or deconstructed. It may be particularly interesting to record those which you had yourself previously taken for granted. In what ways are they 'simultaneously over-simplified, complicated and contradictory'? (Chapter 1, p.12).

COMMENT

In Chapter 1, section 1.2 this exercise was carried out very explicitly for common-sense ideas about poverty. Other examples you may have considered include:

In Chapter 2, Activity 2.1 explored common visual and verbal representations of people with disabilities, showing a range of contradictions. For example, they are commonly seen simultaneously 'as objects of both pity (due to their "cruel fate") and congratulation (for their "cheery fortitude")' (p.50). They are also seen as simultaneously 'a danger or threat to others', and as 'the brave and altruistic "innocent" ' (p.50).

Chapter 3 explored how 'race' is seen as a natural characteristic, so that people can be categorized, ostensibly on the basis of bodily features, into different racial groups. It also explored the way people categorized as black, or as part of a so-called ethnic minority, are seen as different or 'other' and outside of images of the nation. Section 3 showed how 'race relations' in general, and the presence of black children in schools in particular, were taken for granted as constituting problems both in common senses and in academic and policy discussions.

In Chapter 4 a range of common-sense ideas about sexuality were examined. It was suggested that sex was seen as simultaneously private and an object of public discussion; as simultaneously pleasurable and painful, as something sought after and feared. More generally there is a contradiction between views of sex as an expression of natural drives, and as something requiring education and advice, with normative views on the best ways of being sexual.

■ ■ ■

3.1 Personal experience and social science

Can personal experience play a role in social science analyses?

We have suggested that, as social scientists, we have to 'distance ourselves not just from "what everybody knows" but also from what we ourselves "know" about social issues. "What we know" is also part of the "stock of knowledge" in this society' (Chapter 1, p.25). However, Chapters 2, 3 and 4 included examples of how people's personal experiences can be used to illustrate and explore theoretical ideas. What 'we know' from personal experience can also be helpful in questioning the assumptions underlying what is taken for granted, particularly if our own personal experience is out of line with the dominant views. It can become a reference point for a series of questions such as:

- Who is saying this?
- Why are they saying it?
- What are the implications of their views?

Each of the Chapters 2–4 has given examples of how people constructed as 'social problems' (disabled people, black people, gay men and lesbians) have used their experiences to challenge the dominant taken-for-granted views. At the same time, we saw in Chapter 2 (section 6.3) that within the disability movement itself, the role of personal experience is the subject of contestation.

The link between ideas and personal experience has to operate in the other direction too. We can scrutinize our own ideas, by asking ourselves questions such as: what is it that makes me think about these issues in this particular way rather than another? That is, we need to recognize that what we have called our own 'subject position' can lead to particular ways of seeing and interpreting. (We shall consider this again in section 4.1, Activity 5.2.)

We saw in Chapter 2 that the 'taken-for-granted' ideas on disability occur within academic social science as well as in common sense. We have not therefore been arguing that social science offers the objective truth in contrast to subjective personal experience. Chapter 1 argued that the multiple competing perspectives on any issue all make a claim to being the 'correct' account, superior to others, and the 'truth'.

How do we deal with the range of contradictory ideas that have been covered?

We have not been concerned in this book with establishing 'the truth' about any of the topics discussed, or in choosing the 'best' explanations. We want instead to recognize the diverse ways in which social differences and social problems are defined, understood and made sense of, and to show that these different perspectives 'matter' because they have very different consequences. In Chapters 2–4 we have seen that the diverse perspectives are in competition with each other, and that this competition is not an equal one; some constructions are dominant or hegemonic (we shall return to this in section 5). A central task of the chapters in this book has been to show how these constructions and their links to power can be deconstructed.

4   Naturalization of the social

Chapter 1 emphasized that many of the social arrangements and identities in society are so well established that they are taken for granted as common sense and are not even seen as social. Rather, they are assumed to be natural and inevitable, deriving from biology and evolution. This process of attributing taken-for-granted aspects of social arrangements to the realm of nature is described as *naturalization*. Our concern in this book has been to examine 'it's natural' explanations as a form of social construction which 'provides a strong claim to authority and truth, by referring to a world of natural laws that are seen as universal and immutable' (Chapter 1, p.21). So, 'from a social constructionist standpoint, the appearance of the word natural (or unnatural) is usually a warning that deeply embedded patterns of social expectations are at stake' (Chapter 1, p.26).

Ideas of the natural occurred in all three of the central chapters. Let us explore how they appeared, and crucially consider what they tell us about the implications of naturalization of the social.

In Chapter 3 we saw how the physical features of a person's body are used to categorize that person. We pointed out how a physical biological characteristic (skin colour) carries social meanings, but that these are widely seen as natural. Not only is an individual seen as having a 'race', but differences between people based on 'race' are seen as natural as well. Chapter 3 described this as the process of '*racialization*' (section 2.2) and suggested that this immediately has the effect of constructing boundaries between people, so that it becomes possible to leap from physical characteristics to identifying who automatically and rightly belongs to 'the nation'.

Chapter 2 described a variety of ways in which naturalization operates. Dominant views of disability see a person's disability as a characteristic of the individual; disabled people are widely assumed to look different. More generally it is assumed that there is a natural way for disabled people to behave and that they are naturally dependent. Disability is also viewed as 'unnatural' or abnormal, since the natural state of human beings is assumed to be 'able-bodied', a concept that is not seen as being in need of definition. Those who are not able-bodied are therefore disabled or handicapped, and to be pitied or helped. We saw historical changes in these ideas, with disabled people having been seen at certain historical periods as subhuman and hence in need of incarceration or institutionalization. A later approach, described in section 5 of Chapter 2, explores the way in which disability is seen as an unnatural condition or 'illness', and hence in need of treatment by a doctor. This was described as a process of *medicalization.*

Chapter 4 demonstrated the way in which the construction of the 'natural' also constructs what is 'unnatural'. It is widely taken for granted that heterosexuality is natural, and that unnatural sexuality is deviant and in need of control. As in Chapters 2 and 3, we saw how dominant ideas have changed historically. From the late-nineteenth-century sexologists came the idea of homosexuals as a 'third sex', a different type of human subject. This had important consequences not only for how homosexual men and women were seen by others, but also for how they saw themselves, and hence what seemed possible for them in their lives. But in this instance naturalness was used to argue *against* exclusion, as it was also, in a different version, in the 1990s debates on the age of consent for homosexuals (section 5.5). Consideration of this issue also serves to remind us that social constructionism is a perspective and not a politics, so there is no inevitable link between particular constructions of an issue and a political stance. Thus, for example, in the 1990s ideas of a 'gay gene' were used to argue both for the selective abortion of 'gay' foetuses and also for equal rights for gay men and lesbians.

In Chapter 4 we also saw that the existence of prostitution is seen as an inevitable consequence of the natural differences in women's and men's sexuality. As a result, certain questions like 'why do men seek out prostitutes?' are rarely asked, and intervention is directed towards controlling the public manifestations of prostitution, rather than eliminating it.

We can conclude that naturalization helps to 'conceal issues relating to social arrangements and our conventional expectations about them' (Chapter 1, p.28). Deconstructing social arrangements, making them strange, draws attention to aspects of them, including power relations, that are taken for granted and not questioned.

4.1   Essentialism and homogenization

Chapter 1 also introduced the concept of *essentialism*, which was described as 'the belief that social behaviour is determined by some underlying process or "essence" which works itself out in social contexts' (p.28).

In the three subsequent chapters we can find several examples of essentialism. In all cases essentialism implies permanence of a condition or identity which determines people's behaviour and thinking, and the homogenization of people characterized by this essential feature. For example, we saw in Chapter 4 that essentialist accounts may differ, but they share the use of particular categories such as 'heterosexual' and 'homosexual' to describe and group people. People are then assumed not only to differ in terms of their sexual behaviour or practices, but also to be essentially different kinds of people.

Chapter 2 showed how disability is commonly seen as an essential, and hence permanent, characteristic of people, derived from physical/biological/ psychological/ cognitive traits. Chapter 3 presented two different versions of essentialism: first in terms of 'nature', with people's 'race' defined by the physical characteristic of skin colour, and second in terms of 'culture', with people defined as 'ethnic minorities' on the basis of assumed essential characteristics of their 'lifestyles' and ways of behaving.

We have suggested that essentialism implies not only permanence of a condition or identity, but also the homogenization of people defined by this characteristic. Consequently, within an essential category, differences between people are denied. Challenges to this homogenization occurred in all three chapters.

In Chapter 2, Extract 2.5 emphasized 'the complex and varied experiences of disabled people … as, for example, women, sexual beings, private citizens, workers, and so on' (p.50).

Chapter 3 argued that the discourse of 'blackness', although it 'sought to deny the well-established negative associations which the idea of "blackness" carried' (p.118), constructed at the same time an image of a homogeneous black community and experience: 'In this idea of "black" there is no room for members of those ethnic groups assumed to belong to "black" to have a varying range of experiences – they are reduced to a single category' (p.119).

Chapter 4 challenged the idea of a 'unitary phenomenon' of homosexuality (p.175). 'What we have are a multiplicity of feelings, genders, behaviours, identities, relationships, locales, religions, work experiences, reproductive capacities, child-rearing practices, political disagreements, and so forth, that have been appropriated by a few rough categories like "homosexual", "lesbian", "gay" ' (Plummer, 1992, p.14).

5   Social differences and social problems

5.1   Differences, norms and 'othering'

In section 4 we discussed how bodies signal difference, and indicated some consequences of this. Here we want to look further at the issue of difference. People differ in many ways, and we are not seeking to deny those differences. Rather, we wish to emphasize that it is only some differences that are seen as particularly significant, and to consider why those differences are given a special status in common senses, within much social science, and within political and policy debates. The differences that are seen as significant are not only differences in how people look, but in how they behave (such as with hetero-/homosexuality) or in how they live (as with ethnic majority/minority cultures).

The differences we have been considering in this book are all seen in terms of a dichotomy: for example, disabled/able-bodied, white/black, hetero-/homosexual, respectable woman/prostitute. The two sides of this dichotomy are not seen as being of equal value. All these differences are established in relation to a norm, and can only be defined in relation to that norm. So 'disabled' has no meaning for us unless we have a concept of 'able-bodied'; 'black' is defined in relation to white; and homosexuality is defined in opposition to heterosexuality. Chapter 3 described changes in how differences in relation to 'race' have been constructed, and showed the shift from a focus on physical characteristics to a focus on assumptions about how people live, about what is called cultural difference, with only people seen as 'ethnic' having a culture in this sense. In both cases, whether seen as 'race' or 'ethnicity', the categorization of people carries a range of social meanings linked to the power relations that are operating. Thus, 'race' and 'ethnicity' are seen only as characteristics of the minority, subordinated group, and are given meaning in terms of how they are seen as *different from* the supposedly 'unraced' normal majority. In every case it is the 'different' group that is seen as homogeneous and becomes the object of study.

Norms are very powerful because they are taken for granted, not seen as problematic, and not in need of definition. However, if we become 'sceptical strangers', we can ask questions about the meaning of these taken-for-granted terms. We can, in other words, 'problematize' these norms and think about their social meanings, and how these are linked to the power relations that underlie the social arrangements in society.

ACTIVITY 5.2

In order to think about this issue further, try to 'problematize' these norms for yourself. One way of doing this is to consider the following questions:

1   What does 'able-bodied' mean to you?

2   What does 'whiteness' mean to you?

3   What does 'heterosexuality' mean to you?

Since by this stage you have done quite a lot of thinking about these issues, you may find it helpful to ask a friend to answer these questions too.

COMMENT

How you answer these questions is likely to vary according to how you position yourself in the social world, and are positioned by others, in relation to these categories. If you position yourself, or are positioned, in the category defined by the norm, as an 'insider' – that is, as able-bodied, white and/or heterosexual – you may find parts of the exercise quite hard, as it is likely that you are not used to thinking about these taken-for-granted 'normal' categories. You may have found yourself wanting to think about the 'different' or 'other' category because this was much easier.

Alternatively, if you position yourself, or are positioned, as an 'outsider' in the 'other' category in relation to one or more of these differences (as disabled, black/ 'ethnic minority' or as lesbian or gay) then this is likely to affect the meanings you ascribe to them.

Let me give you an example from my own experience, which may help to show both how norms can be theorized and also how personal experience can be used in the dual way described in section 3.1 above: that is, using personal experience to question what is taken for granted, and to consider how what I take for granted is influenced by my subject positions.

In relation to the norms being discussed here, I see myself, and am seen, as an able-bodied, white lesbian, although in some contexts I have choices to keep my sexuality invisible. I am very aware that until recently I had thought much more about heterosexuality than about whiteness or able-bodiedness. I have found, as you may do, that studying social science can challenge ideas that I had held for years.

As someone positioned as an able-bodied person, I do not question, for example, how I will get around physically, whether buildings will be 'accessible', or how I will communicate with others, and I do not generally think of myself as dependent, a characteristic associated with disability. However, consideration of the idea of 'able-bodiedness' and reading the literature from the disability movement, makes me aware that it is as difficult to define 'able-bodied' as it is to define 'disability'. I have also become aware of a range of dependencies that I have in common with most other people, whether able-bodied or disabled. For example, as described in Chapter 2, section 6, I frequently use 'mobility aids' such as cars, buses, trains and planes. I also realize that although I am short-sighted and entirely dependent upon my glasses for carrying out most daily tasks, this is not seen, or experienced by me, as a disability, because my impairment is a very common one, and my sight is relatively easily corrected. As I get older, and my physical capacities (including my eyesight) change, I attribute this to ageing rather than to disablement, although ageing itself is widely constructed as a disabling process.

Reading the accounts of two women walking through two different cities in Chapter 3 (Extracts 3.1 and 3.2) alerted me to differences in my experiences of walking around between the place where I grew up, a white, middle-class London suburb, and the place I live now, a 'multicultural' part of North London. As a child I saw myself, and was positioned by others, as both an insider as a white child, and at the same time as an outsider because my parents were Jewish refugees with 'foreign' accents. The extract by Minnie Bruce-Pratt showed how the particular neighbourhood she lived in, in which she was in a minority numerically, made her conscious of her dominant 'racial' position, as a white person and still privileged.

Living in a multiracial area of London, I am much more conscious of my whiteness now than I was as a child, particularly when interacting with black neighbours and friends, although I am still aware that in most of my daily activities I do not have to think about being white. I am most commonly made aware of it when I am treated differently from black friends, for example when going through customs, and in the way I am rarely asked about my origins, a question frequently posed to people categorized as 'other' racially.

On the other hand, although I see myself clearly as white, I am also aware that, as described in the final section of Chapter 3, 'being white is not enough', and that white people are also racialized (after living in England for over 40 years, my parents were still asked continually about how long they had lived here). Depending upon the particular social context, I also position myself as a racialized subject as a Jewish woman, though not religious, with an understanding from my parents' experiences of the nature of racism. However, it is easier to see myself as 'raced' as Jewish than as white.

Finally, considering heterosexuality, I am much more aware on a daily basis of its position as a dominant norm that excludes me. I am very conscious of ways in which it is taken for granted in everyday discussions of family, marriage and children, even in the way that I am constantly asked whether I am 'Miss' or 'Mrs', and that I don't have an easy or comfortable word for describing my partner, such as 'wife' or 'husband'. It has material consequences in terms of our pension and housing rights. As a category it places me outside it, as different and 'other'. Because of the negative social meanings generally applied to lesbianism, I felt forced when I was younger to ask myself questions about my sexuality such as 'why am I gay?', and to come to terms with being, in the eyes of other people, 'deviant'. I doubt whether many heterosexuals ask themselves about the origins of their heterosexuality.

■ ■ ■

In Chapter 4 there was a brief description of a study of heterosexuality, which demonstrated how people (in this case women) found it difficult to think of themselves as heterosexual. It was something they simply took for granted. Being asked to think about it made them feel uncomfortable, labelled by others rather than able to choose the label for themselves, and cast as 'other'. We also saw in that chapter that heterosexuality is sometimes problematized, for example when it takes a particular form such as 'prostitution', which although conforming (in its heterosexual form) to the dominant norm of heterosexuality, violates gendered norms of 'womanhood'. Thus we saw that in the 1980s it was assumed by people on both sides of the political debate that prostitutes were different from normal women, and in particular excluded from 'motherhood' (Chapter 4, section 5.6).

We have seen that differences are defined in relation to norms, and serve to leave the dominant group as unproblematic, and to place those in the non-dominant, subordinated category as 'other', marginalized and excluded (see Chapter 3, section 3). In the different chapters we have seen many diverse examples of the processes of exclusion. In Chapter 2 we saw how disabled people have at times been excluded from the category 'human', having been regarded as subhuman or lesser human beings. Chapter 3 emphasized the way in which racialization has been used to draw boundaries between people, and to construct 'the nation' as homogeneous and white, thus excluding anyone who does not meet the criteria. Further examples of this can be found in Chapter 4, where opposition to male homosexuality and lesbianism, as well as concern about prostitution, were frequently expressed in racialized terms, with all three of these being seen at various times as a threat to the stability and order of the nation (see Chapter 4, sections 5.4, 6.3 and 6.4). The chapter also argued that lesbian women and women working as prostitutes are excluded from the category 'mother'.

In contrasting 'common senses' and 'social science' we have emphasized that we are not arguing for 'bad' common senses to be replaced by 'good' social science. Social science knowledges are also socially constructed, and need to be subjected to equally rigorous analysis. They frequently incorporate dominant norms implicitly. Chapter 3 gave a good example of this in showing how a specific piece of social science research reflects the 'common association of ethnicity with "non-whiteness"' (p.125). Chapter 2 also pointed out that 'academic knowledge is culpable in contributing to the wider marginalization and distortion of the experiences of disabled people … social scientific knowledge itself is forever contested and subject to controversy' (p.53).

5.2   The social construction of social problems

In each of Chapters 2, 3 and 4, we have seen how those seen as different from the norm are constructed as 'other', become the object of inquiry, and are often seen as deviant and as social problems. We also saw the importance of understanding the social construction of problems within particular socio-historical circumstances. In Chapter 4 it was argued that social constructionism as an approach 'suggests that the meanings given to sexuality vary with specific social and historical circumstances, and that it only has meaning within socio-historical contexts' (p.157).

Chapter 1, section 2 discussed what is 'social' about a social problem, and the assumption that 'something must be done'. Some interesting comparisons and contrasts can be drawn in the way our three examples of social difference, namely disability, 'race' and sexuality, have been socially constructed as problems. It is possible to detect links between particular constructions and solutions.

Although historically it has not always been the case, to a large extent disabled people are seen as *having problems*, through no fault of their own, and hence requiring care to assist them in daily living. In contrast, in Chapter 3 we saw how black children, in sufficient numbers, were seen in the 1960s as *being a problem* for white, 'native' children in schools. This basic supposition was not questioned, even though the way the problem was constructed (from ideas about assimilation to integration and multiculturalism), and hence the proposed solutions, did change. However, in Chapter 3 there were also examples of so-called ethnic minority children being seen as having problems, though this was expressed in the language of 'needs'. For example, the Swann Report referred to the 'particular educational needs which an ethnic minority pupil may have, arising for example from his or her linguistic or cultural background' (Chapter 3, p.115).

In Chapter 4 we saw that at different historical times lesbians, gay men and women working as prostitutes have predominantly been seen as *being problems* that need to be legally controlled. An exception to this was in the debates around the 1967 law reforms on male homosexuality, in which those arguing for reform constructed homosexual men as *having a problem*: homosexuality for them was very much a form of disability to be pitied and, where possible, treated.

Chapter 4 also demonstrated the importance of gender in constructing social problems linked to sexuality. For example, lesbians and gay men are seen as very different kinds of problems requiring different kinds of solutions, and in relation to prostitution it has been clear that it is the women working as prostitutes who are seen as the problem rather than the men who seek out and use their services.

More generally, Chapter 4 highlighted the importance of *morality* in constructing social problems related to sexuality. Thus, for example, Smart (1995) argued that 'prostitution' is essentially a *moral* category (section 5.6). In relation to homosexuality, although medical discourses largely replaced religious discourses at the end of the nineteenth century, the latter survived throughout the twentieth century, with homosexuality continuing to be constructed by some commentators, and in many common senses, as a sin or vice in which people choose to indulge. Homosexuality is therefore seen as not just unnatural but also abnormal and immoral. People are condemned because they are seen as choosing to behave in an abnormal way. This is in contrast to being disabled or part of a particular 'racial group', both of which are seen as characteristics over which the individual has no choice.

This does not mean that morality is irrelevant to discussions of disability and 'race'. We saw in Chapter 2, for example, that in the Old Testament 'the moral censure against disability is extremely strong' (p.59), with disability being seen as a punishment from God. The chapter showed links between this idea and the construction of HIV as a punishment for immorality by gay men. You will also be familiar with common-sense ideas about the 'cultural' patterns of some groups of people described as ethnic minorities who are frequently seen as less moral, particularly in relation to marriage and having children, and as more likely to be criminal. These sets of ideas are applied particularly to people described as 'Afro-Caribbean' or 'West Indian'.

Chapter 4 also demonstrated how the distinction between 'public' and 'private' is important in the way in which social problems are constructed, particularly those linked to sexuality. The social reforms of the 1950s and 1960s in relation to prostitution and male homosexuality were justified on the grounds that the law should intervene as little as possible in the 'private' lives of individuals. This distinction between public and private is one that many of you may have taken for granted. However, analysis of these legal reforms showed that this distinction is itself a social construction. For consenting adult gay men a hotel room was defined as a public place, and for women working as prostitutes, sitting in their window was constructed as being 'in the street' (see Chapter 4, sections 6.3 and 5.5).

In the discussions in this book we have also seen links between the various aspects of difference. In particular, Chapter 4 showed how constructions of sexuality are intersected by social differences related to 'race' and disability, as well as to other differences such as gender, class and age. In Chapter 2 we saw the links that were made in the early twentieth century between people with learning difficulties and so-called 'primitive ethnic groups', who, it was taken for granted, were naturally inferior (section 5.2). In Chapter 4 we saw how some gay men and lesbians have likened being gay to having a distinct 'ethnicity' and have tried to argue for a minority ethnic status that is deserving of greater recognition and rights. It is not uncommon for those who are black or seen as members of an ethnic minority to be described in terms of having a 'handicap' or 'disability', as if to emphasize that this is something for which someone cannot be blamed, but should be pitied. Interestingly, in Extract 3.4 from the Institute of Race Relations in Chapter 3, which challenged dominant constructions of multicultural education in the 1980s, the experiences of black children in schools were also described in terms of 'disabilities', though in this case not ones produced by nature but by 'the racialist attitudes and the racist practices in the larger society and in the educational system itself' (Chapter 3, p.114). You may wish to reflect on this in relation to the social model of disability.

6 Contestation and power

Throughout this book we have emphasized that everything is contested, whether it is the definition of a topic, the nature of the problem, or ideas on how to solve it. Crucially, we have seen that the contests are not ones between equals – some constructions, whether described as labels, ideologies or discourses, are hegemonic (see Chapter 1, section 6.2): that is, they are unquestioningly regarded as being the truth, whether through being accepted as 'common sense', or seen as 'expert knowledge'.

6.1 Discourses and social intervention

Chapter 1 suggested that when we are considering social issues and problems, the idea of *discourses* is an important one. Discourses are described as 'ways of organizing knowledge. They define what the problem is; they say what is worth knowing and what can be said. They produce the "norms" against which deviation or abnormality is marked … [they] shape and become institutionalized in social policies and the organizations through which they are carried out' (Chapter 1, p.35).

Chapter 1 therefore suggested that discourses have the following characteristics:

- They define the nature of the problem.
- They shape what is worth knowing, and what constitutes 'truth'.
- They are institutionalized within social arrangements and relations of power.

As an example Chapter 1 described the way in which discourses of poverty shape what can be said about poverty, whether in everyday conversations, academic research or political debate, and how these discourses have been and continue to be institutionalized in social arrangements such as the workhouse, charity organizations, benefit offices, means tests, etc. Such discourses are also institutionalized in relations of power, so that 'in relation to poverty, they empower … state agencies to monitor, assess or intervene in the lives of poor people' (Chapter 1, p.36).

It is because competing perspectives share a definition of the problem that they can compete and argue. Perspectives that start somewhere else, or do not share the definition of the problem, have great difficulty in 'making themselves heard' or understood. They do not fit the terms of reference of the discourse. An example of this can be found in Chapter 4, which described the difficulty that campaigners against child prostitution were having in their struggle. Their proposed solutions derived from a different definition of the problem as one of child abuse, a discourse that could not be heard in the context of debates on prostitution.

Chapter 2 offered a 'clear illustration of the complex intertwining of social constructions and specific policy interventions' (p.76). It showed how a particular 'expert' discourse, that of the medical profession, came to 'own' the problems of 'mental illness' and 'mental deficiency', and how these discourses constructed the problem of disability in individualistic terms as a product of bodily or mental defect or impairment creating vulnerability and dependence, and hence requiring medical intervention to deal with this apparently natural state. The chapter went on to argue that these medical policies and practices helped to 'solidify' these individualizing discourses which in turn informed the anti-discrimination legislation of the mid 1990s.

6.2   Processes of contestation

To a large extent in this chapter, as in Chapters 2, 3 and 4, I have been referring to the dominant or hegemonic sets of ideas about disability, 'race' and sexualities. However, the three central chapters also considered the challenges to these discourses that have come from social movements concerned with struggles against disablism, racism and heterosexism, and for the rights of their constituent groups. In each case these groups challenged the discourses that organized the knowledge about these issues, and which were institutionalized in laws, social policies and the medical, educational and legal practices. It was also shown in each case that these new discourses themselves resulted in contradictions.

ACTIVITY 5.3

Look back over Chapters 2, 3 and 4 and identify examples of the role of social movements in the struggle over constructions of problems. Note in particular any contradictions that can arise.

COMMENT

Chapter 4 showed how, at the end of the nineteenth century, the very process of categorizing people as heterosexual or homosexual did not just construct new homosexual subjects who could be controlled legally. For the first time particular kinds of people who saw themselves as 'homosexuals' were able to organize with others who shared their subject position, to resist the legal controls, and to campaign for changes in the law. The trial over *The Well of Loneliness*, it was suggested, had a similar effect for lesbians. In the late 1960s new gay subjects were produced for the first time who organized in a different way and demanded a different set of rights, and to be included as people in relationships who could have equal rights with heterosexuals in relation to 'marriage' and parenthood. At the same time we saw how this new discourse homogenized gay people, denying differences between them, and denying the possibilities of change or of bisexuality.

In Chapter 3 we saw how the discourse of 'blackness', which developed out of struggles against racism, nevertheless homogenized black people as a single category, denying them diversity of experiences. It was argued that the 'anti-racist education' perspective not only 'excluded from its view those black people whose experiences were structured by more than just racism – by gender or sexuality for example … it excluded white groups whose experiences were also structured by processes of racialization' (Chapter 3, p.119). Through the case study of the Burnage Report, we saw how a particular set of social constructions of 'race' and 'racism' served to exclude white people from involvement in the development of anti-racist policies in the school, whilst having no impact on the 'wider structure of racial exclusions found outside the school' (p.124).

Chapter 2 described how the dominant view of the social problem of disability was challenged by the disability movement of the 1980s and 1990s, which defined the problem in a very different way. Their view was that people's problems are caused by a disabling society which is organized to meet the needs of so-called able-bodied people. However, in section 6.3 of that chapter we saw how this model has itself been challenged from within the disability movement, both for privileging personal experience as a form of evidence and argument, and also for denying differences in the personal experiences of being disabled. As in Chapters 3 and 4, we saw how the discourses that challenge the hegemony of the dominant discourses themselves result in homogenizing disabled people, denying other differences such as those related to gender, 'race', sexuality, age and class.

■ ■ ■

7   The consequences of social constructions

Throughout this book we have been emphasizing that social constructions are not just interesting sets of ideas which generate academic argument, but that on the contrary they have very real consequences for people's lives.

What kind of consequences have been identified?

The consequences of constructions have been discussed in terms of:

■ How people see themselves and understand their own experience; what choices or options they feel they have; and how they are seen by others (their subjectivities and subject positions).

■ The extent to which people are included or excluded from a range of social relationships and activities or from imaginary groupings such as 'the nation'.

■ The way in which they are embedded in concrete policies and practices which in turn reinforce (or solidify) the social construction on which they are based.

There are many examples in all the chapters. For instance, Chapter 1, section 8.1 looked at some of the organizing principles of the discourse of poverty and their consequences.

Chapter 3 argued that the social construction of 'racial groups', whether in terms of physical characteristics of bodies ('races') or as ways of living ('ethnicities') have a wide range of 'real life' effects: 'they help organize and give meaning to the interactions between people who are "known" as "racial" or "ethnic" and those who are not known in this way' (Chapter 3, p.135).

In addition, through the discussion of multicultural and anti-racist education, Chapter 3 provided detailed examples of the way in which social constructions are embedded in social policies, whether these policies are in line with the dominant ideas in society or aim to challenge them. Finally, the examination of the Burnage Report showed the two-way relationship between social policies and social constructions. Thus, the policies aimed at dealing with the 'problems' of 'social difference' were built upon the bits of common sense about 'racial groups' and 'social differences' described above. In turn, these policies contributed to the construction of these as 'real' differences, both natural and inevitable.

Chapters 2 and 4 also both looked at the changing ways in which particular groups of people (disabled people, gay men, lesbians, women working as prostitutes) are constructed as 'other', as different from the assumed normal group. They described some of the consequences of this in terms of how people see themselves, and are seen by others, for the options and choices they feel (or others assume) they have in their lives, and for their capacity to organize against discrimination. Like Chapter 3, these chapters demonstrated clear links between these social constructions and social policies. Some of them have been referred to in this review chapter, but you may wish to look back at these chapters to identify these links in more detail. Both chapters also give examples of the way discourses (medical and legal in particular) literally gave power to, or empowered, professionals to act, whether to 'treat' disabled people or homosexuals, or to caution 'common prostitutes'.

8   Conclusion

The chapters in this book have taken you on a journey from ideas that are very familiar – 'what everybody knows' – to new and different ways of trying to make sense of the social world in which we live. This has involved engaging with some quite difficult and probably new concepts, as well as with material that may have personal and emotional resonance, and which on occasions may have been quite disturbing or painful. It is likely that you have had some of your own 'taken-for-granted' ideas challenged, and this too can be quite difficult, but also exciting.

Let us consider how this approach might be adopted in relation to another social issue. In the 1980s and 1990s many discussions of social welfare focused on ideas of 'the family', and fears of its break-up. This was seen in the UK by many social commentators and politicians of both main political parties as an indication of a social crisis and a threat to the social order and stability of society. Particular concerns were raised about the increase in the number of lone-parent families, as well as about people living openly as lesbian and gay couples, particularly with children, or as 'travellers'. Adopting a social constructionist approach would lead us to examine the assumptions underlying such views, and to see that they are based on the taken-for-granted idea that a particular family form is the 'best', because it is 'natural'.

If we adopt a social constructionist approach we would proceed to ask questions about the history of such ideas, to look at how 'family' is defined, and to recognize that there are competing definitions of 'family'. We would consider how the dominant discourses of the family have been embedded in social policy and legislation in relation to families; how these discourses have given the power to state agencies to intervene in families, or in certain kinds of families; and how these policies and practices have in turn helped 'particular ways of thinking and acting become "habits", institutionalized and "sedimented" as the normal way of life' (Chapter 1, p.40). The specific examples explored in this book might also alert you to consider what kinds of living arrangements are viewed as 'family' and the extent to which people who are 'othered' in terms of disability, 'race' and sexuality are included or excluded by discourses of the 'normal family'. To read more on these issues in relation to the family, see **Lentell (1998)** and **Hall (1998)**.

Although in this book we have applied the social constructionist approach to particular aspects of social difference, we have throughout emphasized its general applicability to the study of the social world. In your further reading or study of social differences, social welfare and social policy, you will find all sorts of ideas that are taken for granted in both common senses and within policy debates. We hope that you now feel better equipped to question both the taken-for-granted statements of others – whether expressed as 'common sense', academic social science, medical or legal 'expertise', statements of policy or justifications of those policies by politicians – and also the challenges to the dominant positions by pressure groups or social movements.

References

Hall, C. (1998) 'A family for nation and empire', in Lewis, G. (ed.) *Forming Nation, Framing Welfare*, London, Routledge in association with The Open University.

Lentell, H. (1998) 'Families of meaning: contemporary discourses of the family', in Lewis, G. (ed.) *Forming Nation, Framing Welfare*, London, Routledge in association with The Open University.

Plummer, K. (1992) 'Speaking its name: inventing a gay and lesbian studies', in Plummer, K. (ed.) *Modern Homosexualities*, London, Routledge.

Smart, C. (1995) *Law, Crime and Sexuality*, London, Sage.

Acknowledgements

Grateful acknowledgement is made to the following sources for permission to reproduce material in this book:

Text

Chapter 2: 'The best of British – Phil fights deafness to lead chess challenge', *Haringey Weekly Herald and North London Advertiser*, 10 January 1990, North London Newspapers; Roderick, C. (1987) '27 years of hell – and he's still smiling', *Star Sunday Sport*, 27 September 1987; the extract by Pam Evans reprinted on pp.48–9 is from *Pride Against Prejudice: Transforming Attitudes to Disability* by Jenny Morris, first published by The Women's Press Ltd, 1991, 34 Great Sutton Street, London EC1V 0DX, and is used by permission of The Women's Press Ltd; Humphries, S. and Gordon, P. (1992) *Out of Sight: The Experience of Disability 1900–1950*, Northcote House Publishers Ltd; Keith, L. 'Tomorrow I am going to re-write the English language', *Able Lives*, © Spinal Injuries Association; ***Chapter 3:*** Boyle, E. (1963) 'Speech to House of Commons', *Hansard*, 25 November–6 December 1963. Parliamentary copyright material is reproduced with the permission of the Controller of Her Majesty's Stationery Office on behalf of Parliament; ***Chapter 4:*** Quinn, S. (1996) 'Women's power a "turn-off"', *The Guardian*, 16 April 1996, © *The Guardian*.

Photographs/Illustrations

p.7: (top) Tom Jenkins; (bottom) Peter Marshall/Photofusion; *p.11:* Crispin Hughes/Photofusion; *p.18:* Michael Abrahams/Network; *p.22:* David Hoffman; *p.23:* Neil Libbert/Network; *p.27:* (top) Mo Wilson/Format; (bottom right) Bob Watkins/Photofusion; (bottom left) Hulton-Deutsch Collection; *p.29:* Vaughan Melzer Photography; *p.36:* Harry Venning; *p.48:* Mary Evans Picture Library; *p.51:* Tom Roberts © 1987; *p.62: Brothers and Sisters*, no.538, January 1938; *p.63:* (top) Barnardo's Photographic Archive; (bottom) London Metropolitan Archives; *p.66:* (left) Scope; (right) Mencap; *p.81:* Mark Tew © 1995; *p.83:* © David Hevey/Camerawork/Joseph Rowntree Foundation; *p.100:* (top left) Virginia R. Domínguez (1994) *White by Definition*, Rutgers University Press; (top right) Barbara Tizard and Ann Phoenix (1993) *Black, White or Mixed Race?*, Routledge. Photo: Lucy Tizard. Design: Andrew Corbett; (bottom) Henry Louis Gates Jr (1994) *Colored People*, Penguin Books Ltd. Photo: FPG/Robert Harding Picture Library; *p.113:* Murdo MacLeod/*The Guardian*; *p.144:* The Advertising Archives; *p.154:* (top) © Kippa Matthews; (bottom) The Advertising Archives; *p.166:* Mary Evans Picture Library; *p.170:* The Hulton-Deutsch Collection; *p.180:* The Hulton-Deutsch Collection; *p.183:* Paul Lowe/Network.

Figures

Figures 2.1 and 2.2: courtesy of the Scottish Equality Awareness Trainers in Disability.

Tables

Table 2.1: Lonsdale, S. (1990) *Women and Disability: The Experience of Physical Disability among Women*, Macmillan Press Ltd; *Table 3.1:* Klein, R. (1995) 'Where prejudice still flares into violence', *Times Educational Supplement*, 6 January 1995, © Times Newspapers Ltd 1995.

Index

The Open University Course Team

The Open University

Melanie Bayley	*Editor*
Ann Boomer	*Discipline Secretary*
David Calderwood	*Project Controller*
Hilary Canneaux	*Course Manager*
John Clarke	*Author/Course Team Chair*
Allan Cochrane	*Author*
Lene Connolly	*Print Buyer*
Troy Cooper	*Author*
Nigel Draper	*Editor*
Ross Fergusson	*Author*
Sharon Gewirtz	*Reading Member*
Peggotty Graham	*Reading Member*
Fiona Harris	*Editor*
Rich Hoyle	*Graphic Designer*
Gordon Hughes	*Author and Editor, Books 4 and 5*
Jonathan Hunt	*Co-publishing Co-ordinator*
Maggie Hutchinson	*Reading Member*
Sue Lacey	*Secretary*
Mary Langan	*Author and Editor, Book 3*
Patti Langton	*Producer, BBC/OUPC*
Helen Lentell	*Author*
Gail Lewis	*Author and Editor, Books 2 and 4*
Vic Lockwood	*Producer, BBC/OUPC*
Lilian McCoy	*Author*
Eugene McLaughlin	*Author*
John Muncie	*Author/Co-Course Team Chair*
Pam Owen	*Graphic Artist*
Doreen Pendlebury	*Secretary*
Sharon Pinkney	*Author*
Esther Saraga	*Author and Editor, Book 1*
Paul Smith	*Liaison Librarian/Picture Researcher*
Pauline Turner	*Course and Discipline Secretary*

External Contributors

Marian Barnes	*Author, Health Services Management Centre, University of Birmingham*
Janet English	*Tutor Panel, Region 11, The Open University*
Ian Gazeley	*Author, School of Social Sciences, University of Sussex*
Catherine Hall	*Author, Department of Sociology, University of Essex*
Mary J. Hickman	*Author, Irish Studies Centre, University of North London*
Eluned Jeffries	*Tutor Panel, Region 02, The Open University*
Chris Jones	*External Assessor, Professor of Social Work, University of Liverpool*
Gerry Mooney	*Author, Department of Applied Social Studies, University of Paisley*
Lydia Morris	*Author, Department of Sociology, University of Essex*
Janet Newman	*Author, School of Public Policy, University of Birmingham*
Lynne Poole	*Tutor Panel, Region 11, The Open University*
Pat Thane	*Author, School of Social Sciences, University of Sussex*

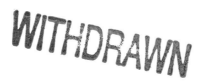